Surviving Lupus, Levaquin, & Life!

Surviving Lupus, Levaquin, & Life!

Healing Brokenness with Faith, Gratitude, & Praying Through Pliés

RHONDA JEAN BOLTON

Expanded 2nd Edition of Praying Through Pliés

Photography and design by Stan Bolton

DEDICATION

With Deepest Love & Gratitude to My Husband,
Stan Bolton

In Loving Memory of My Mother
Colleene Thornton Short, My Father, William Robert
Short, and My Cousin, Dea Busic Cox

ACKNOWLEDGMENTS

With Special Thanksgiving for Contributions of Time, Talent, Prayers, and Unfailing Support from

My family
Children Jeff Hall & Laurie H. Heavner, Ashley B. Lamb, and grandchildren, Preston, Natalie, & Gretchen Heavner, AB & Jack Lamb, and my aunts, Carolyn Baker & Mickey Price, and my cousin, Judy Kirkland, whose ideas and suggestions proved invaluable

My friends
Barbara Barringer, Jen Boggs, Leia Hamlyn, Roxy Linderman, Gail McCombs, Linda Nachtigall, Jenny Propst, Fran Speer, John Thomas, and Gretchen Wilson

The Mind, Body, & Spirit Class of First Presbyterian Church, Morganton, NC
Diane Clark, Susan Duckworth, Anita Hodges, LaNelle Jennings, Mary Lou McDaniel, Sandra Morton, and Jane Tate

My friends and proofreaders
Lena Hardaway and Lori Murray

My friend
Fran Coffey for her reassurance and formatting savvy

My marketing advisor
Ben Willis: Director of the Small Business Center at Caldwell Community College, Hudson, NC whose enthusiasm and mentoring fanned the creative fires

My Healthcare Providers
Garland Hughes, MD, for whom a thank you could never
be enough
Andrew Laster, MD, whose skilled and compassionate
care keeps the flares in remission
The therapists of Healthy at Home: Carolinas HealthCare
System Blue Ridge who helped me believe that I could
achieve my goals

My Spiritual Supporters and friends
Reverend Karla Woggan and The Episcopal Church of the
Ascension, Hickory, NC
Staff & Congregation of First Presbyterian Church,
Morganton NC
Robert Smith, who encouraged me to include my
miraculous epilogue
Reverend Michael Bailey

Blair Abee, who provided ample suggestions and
resources

And with Lifelong Gratitude for
The Louis Nunnery School of Ballet, where I learned to
plié

Table of Contents

Preface ____ 9

Beginnings _______________________________________ 13

Choices ____ 16

Gratitude _______________________________________ 21

Exercise ____ 25

Sleep____ 35

Stress and Relaxation _____________________________ 40

Nutrition____ 47

Neurotoxicity & the Nervous System __________________ 53

Levaquin____ 57

The First Year: July 2015-June 2016 __________________ 67

The Second Year: June 2016-June 2017 ________________ 84

The Third Year: June 2017-June 2018 _________________ 93

The Fourth Year: June 2018-June 2019_________________ 98

Epilogue ____ 107

Fluoroquinolone Antibiotics:The Facts_________________ 111

Living a Healthy Lifestyle ___________________________ 116

Choices and Gratitude_____________________________ 118

Gratitude Journaling ______________________________ *119*

Rejoice ______________________________ *120*

Miracles ______________________________ *121*

Finding Your Pliés ______________________________ *122*

The Morning Readings ______________________________ *124*

About the Author ______________________________ *127*

Preface

Make sickness itself a prayer. Saint Francis de Sales

In June of 2019, I danced again! Really danced. In a ballet. On a stage. With no one physically supporting me. Without a mirror to tell me whether I was upright—or beginning to fall. Sharing a stage again with granddaughters whose smiles were louder than any applause!

My prayer was that my brain would remember four minutes of choreography, and that my legs would last for those same four minutes. And for four miraculous minutes, I danced with joy, gratitude, and no small amount of astonishment! Because four years earlier, in June of 2015, I wasn't sure I would walk again, or even live.

My journey of survival, however, began long before June of 2015. I was diagnosed with lupus several decades ago. After being asked numerous times how I dealt with this condition so well, I decided to share my journey by writing a book in hopes that someone reading it would find inspiration and encouragement as well as easy-to-follow suggestions for dealing with chronic and life-changing conditions.

The catalyst and foundation for this book was a poem that I had written called "Praying Through Pliés," but life was busy, and I never seemed to have time to write. An antibiotic called Levaquin then dealt me a blow that complicated and changed my health and life dramatically. Being unable to return to work, I certainly had the time to write!

My initial outline and introduction complete, I started to simply continue writing my book as planned, but I realized that not only had my path taken a totally different turn, but that this second part needed to be told as well. While I continue to hope that you find inspiration and encouragement within these pages, I am equally committed to educate about the possible dangers of prescription medication.

First there was lupus, then the devastating reaction to Levaquin. Both conditions are and will continue to be part of my journey. They have been life-altering and transformative. Through it all, my mantra has remained the same: I call it praying through plies.

Why this particular mantra? Pliés, by making it possible to transition from one step to the next, are the foundation of ballet. My mantra focuses on the sequence of pliés that are done at the beginning of barre work, the beginning of a ballet class. A lifelong student of ballet, this muse captivated my soul at a young age, and the joy that ballet brought has carried me throughout my life. During times of loss and grief, and during times of illness, it brought me home. This is my story of living with chronic illness, and the power of praying through plies.

Dance, when you're broken open… Rumi

plié
\ *plē- ˈā* \ : *a bending of the knees.*
Plies often begin barre work, signaling the beginning of the
ballet class. As the body rises and descends slowly, the arms flow
gracefully, creating a sense of floating with the music.

<h1 style="text-align:center">Praying through Pliés</h1>

When I take the barre,
The tightness melts, and pain barely whispers.
My body lifts, a subtle cue signaling transformation
And I am a young girl again.

Legs gently bending,
Graceful strength flowing through my arms,
An ageless time traveler returning home.
Following a cadence centuries old.

As healing energy and affirmations
embrace my very cells,
The dance begins, I am whole,
And I pray through pliés.

Prayers filled with gratitude
To all who have made this moment possible,
Thanking God and my body
For one more time at the barre.

As decades of my muscle memory engage,
Rhythmic ritual becomes a meditation,
Focus sharpens to a stillpoint,
And I pray through pliés.

Slow, lovely notes flow.
My eyes glance heavenward,
I am mindful only of this moment,
And I pray through plies.

1

Beginnings

... behind all your stories is always your mother's story, because hers is where yours begins." Mitch Albom, <u>For One More Day</u>

Johns Hopkins defines autoimmunity as a condition that occurs when the immune system goes awry and attacks the body and its own healthy tissues. Autoimmune diseases cannot be cured. Classified as chronic conditions, they typically follow periods of remissions and exacerbations, or flares. Often, there is a genetic link. In general, they are managed by following a treatment plan that includes medication, a proper diet, exercise, and avoiding stress.

Lupus is an autoimmune disease that can perceive any cell, organ, or system in the body as a foreign invader. It then attempts to destroy the enemy. It can mimic many other conditions and often baffles healthcare providers. As with most chronic conditions, the severity, treatment, and the prognosis can vary from person to person. Since it affects so many body systems, symptoms can vary over the course of this disease—sometimes on a day-to-day basis.

Depending on the individual, flares can occur seemingly without reason or because of exposure to a triggering event. Triggers such as illness, stress, allergens, or exposure to toxic substances are also quite individual in nature.

Lupus was the diagnosis I received in my 30's. As it evolved like a chameleon of sorts, it often looked like a mixture of connective tissue disorders. Thyroid dysfunction and Raynaud's Syndrome, a condition where the circulation in the hands and feet is impaired, had an early onset, while vasculitis, pericarditis, and pleuritis, the inflammation of blood vessels and the linings around the heart and lungs, would come and go over the years. Pain in joints and muscles has been present since the beginning, but the degree of discomfort varies widely. Mysterious fevers and flu-like symptoms may appear and just as suddenly, disappear.

Although dry eyes, nose, and mouth were also early symptoms, they became worse as I reached my 60's, and even with frequent use of artificial tears, I began to have small lacerations on my eyes. Along with prescription medication for dry eyes and a humidifier, I also had to use mineral-oil eye drops at night to prevent damage. Nasal spray, in a saline gel formula, and mouth lozenges that adhered to the roof of the mouth, releasing moisture over a period of hours, were daily necessities. After further diagnostic work and evaluation of all symptoms, I received an additional diagnosis of a second autoimmune diagnosis: Sjogren's Syndrome with other organ involvement.

I had watched my mother struggle for decades with Sjogren's and Scleroderma, yet another autoimmune disease. Our lab abnormalities and our medical journeys were remarkably similar. She became disabled in her 40's, and she died at age 64 — six weeks after being diagnosed with non-Hodgkin's Lymphoma. I learned later that there is an elevated risk for developing malignancies, especially non-Hodgkin's Lymphoma, with autoimmune disease and especially with Sjogren's Syndrome.

A strong and courageous individual, my mother rarely complained. I could sometimes hear her crying in the bathroom when she changed the bandages on the painful, gaping wounds on her legs caused by vasculitis from the scleroderma. When she was dying, she refused hospice care because she didn't want to stop chemotherapy. She didn't want the message she left to be one of giving in to any disease. She was truly valiant!

I like to think—at least I hope—that I inherited her backbone and her grace as well. Her journey and her model of strength taught me that I must take control of my journey by empowering myself and by not giving in to a disease. Wisdom, hope, and courage I learned from my mother, and I added a few insights to this mix as I traveled my journey. One of these was the meditative mantra that I called praying through plies. A prayer filled with gratitude that began at a ballet class would soon encompass all the aspects of my healing journey. Praying through pliés would become the lovely metaphor that filled my days.

...When I take the barre,
The tightness melts, and pain barely whispers.
My body lifts, a subtle cue signaling transformation
And I am a young girl again...

2
Choices

Everything can be taken from a man but one thing: the last of the human freedoms — to choose one's attitude in any given set of circumstances, to choose one's own way. Victor Frankl

What do you do when you're dealt a bad gene, a card that has the potential to change your life, perhaps even destroy it? As I see it, you have some choices, for ultimately it is your choice. You didn't choose this disease, this obstacle, but you can choose how you will perceive it. The following are ways that I perceived my disease over the years. While these first two perceptions seemed more like reactions than choices at the time, I later realized that I did indeed choose them!

- *Helplessness*: By giving your condition the power, the control, you have given up and will probably choose whatever gives you immediate satisfaction and comfort. After all, it can't be cured, so does it really matter what you do or don't do?
- *Getting angry and remaining stuck there*: Your valuable and limited energy is used to fight every loss, every symptom, and every challenge.
- *Embracing:* This disease is a part of you, a part that is confused and a little crazy, but nonetheless a part of you. You may try to learn what it has to teach you. This is a much healthier choice than the first two, but transformation won't happen here!
- *Being grateful:* This is where transformation begins!

Yes, I said grateful! For me, it was a lengthy process. You will probably think about the other choices first — the giving up, the anger, the embracing. You might even live with one for a short time - or permanently. You yell, "Why me?" You cry, you deny, you grapple. You process the changes. You imagine your life's map, and you look at all the possible outcomes, and all the possible consequences. After all the layers peel away, you eventually surrender. The war is over.

This is the turning point! Now is the moment you make the decision that will determine your future. You look at your body, your mind, and your spirit, and ask "What am I going to do with this?" You begin to choose how you will live with this passenger and how it will color, shape, and weave your life's fabric from this moment on.

Getting to this turning point, reaching the decision that I would choose gratitude, took many, many years. As a psychiatric mental health nurse and licensed counselor, I know that our thoughts are powerful tools of healing, and our physical, emotional, and spiritual beings listen to our thoughts. John Milton said that the mind is its own place, and in itself, can make a Heaven of Hell, a Hell of Heaven, so be careful what you choose to think! Be very careful what message you choose, because our thoughts not only have the power to heal — they have the power to damage our minds, bodies, and spirits.

Faith decided my choice. "Rejoice always, in everything, give thanks" from 1 Thessalonians 5:16, 18, began to resonate deep within my brokenness. Rejoice always, every minute, of every day, and in everything — not just during the good times, the sunny days, and in the joy of family, but during the dark days. During the devastation of grief and the time of illness, give thanks.

I chose to rejoice. I chose gratitude. It hasn't always been simple or easy. There are dark days. There is grief. There is illness. Times when another piece is lost, a thread broken. Some can be found, mended. Other pieces, simply gone.

How? How do I feel gratitude toward an illness that limits and alters my life goals, an illness that can be painful and destructive? Because it changed my life and confirmed that our time here is short. It made me realize that nothing is guaranteed, that people that I love need to be told now, that all of those things that I love, the things that I said I would make time for someday, need to be done now!

One of my "somedays" was ballet. We had a fragmented but lengthy history together. I began studying ballet at age 5 and continued regularly until around age 13 when I stopped because of an injury. I could have returned to class the next year but chose not to because I was afraid that I was too far behind. The teenage years and high school passed. Although I hadn't returned to my ballet school, the living room floor became my stage, and a high-back chair was a perfect barre. My former ballet instructor welcomed students of all ages including adults, and at age 20, and newlywed, I bought new pointe shoes and called him. One year later, I had just been asked to be a member of the ballet company when I learned that I was pregnant. Within two years, I was a mother of two. The pointe shoes retired once again, and a different floor and chair became my dance studio for the next 20 years. I always knew I would return one day. I was 42 when my mother died. With grief came the realization that "someday" was now.

...Legs gently bending,
Graceful strength flowing through my arms,
An ageless time traveler returning home.
Following a cadence centuries old....

I would return to ballet without thought of being too old, of being behind. I would return with rejoicing, and gratitude! Gratitude to this disease for reminding me to do that which I love before it is too late. Gratitude for each moment that finds me at the barre.

This is when I began the practice of praying through pliés, praying as I rejoiced. Beginning each class and every home practice with a moving prayer of gratitude that healed my body, mind, and spirit.

Health and wholeness do not necessarily mean there is absence of disease! Wholeness is a state of being, a place within where there is peace, hope, and appreciation for the gifts you've been given. You cradle yourself deeply within your heart, sending messages of love, of wholeness, of appreciation with each heartbeat. The seeds have been planted, and transformation will begin!

Transformation is more than just awareness or a new way of thinking and perceiving. While our thoughts and perceptions are critical for true and lasting wholeness, it also requires a commitment to care for yourself. Along with practicing gratitude to strengthen and nourish your spirit, you promise yourself that you will do all that is within your power and current situation to give this miraculous, glorious gift - your body - all that it needs to become as healthy and vibrant as possible. This promise involves taking an honest look at your lifestyle and making needed changes in the areas of diet, exercise, rest, and stress management.

We are not immortal. Perhaps you can't cure your disease, but you can transform your perception of its effect on your life. Knowing that you have done all you can do brings empowerment, peace, and wholeness of mind, body, and spirit! And then you pray prayers of gratitude. God will do the rest.

How we choose what we do, and how we approach it…will determine whether the sum of our days adds up to a formless blur, or to something resembling a work of art.
Mihaly Csikszentmihalyi

3

Gratitude

*If the only prayer you ever say in your entire life is thank you,
it will be enough. Meister Eckhart*

In Chapter 2, I talked about choosing gratitude and how it altered my perception of my illness, but in this brief chapter, I wanted to give you some easy suggestions about how to practice a gratitude-filled life. There has been an awareness of the relationship between health and gratitude for thousands of years. In a physical sense, grateful people often have stronger immune systems, perhaps because they often live a healthy lifestyle. Emotionally, those who practice gratitude seem to enjoy a more positive mood and experience less anxiety and depression. It even helps some people sleep better!

Living a life of gratitude is a simple habit to create. Steps to creating a gratitude-based life are as easy as beginning and ending each day by mentally listing 5 things for which you are grateful. It is even more powerful when these things are written in a gratitude journal. This journal can be an inexpensive school composition notebook or a special writing book with blank pages and pictures that inspire you. Commit to trying this for 2 months: you should see significant changes in your life!

Commit is the key word. It takes effort to change any habit but especially one that involves changing your thinking. Thoreau said it well:

As a single footstep will not make a path on the earth, so a single thought will not make a pathway in the mind. To make a deep physical path, we walk again and again. To make a deep mental path, we must think over and over the kind of thoughts we wish to dominate our lives.

As you choose your thoughts, you are ultimately choosing who you are and who you will become. Let me repeat that statement: you have the power to choose who you are right now and who you will become!

In order to live a life of gratitude, you must choose thoughts of gratitude! The brain can only think one thought and process one thought at a time, so let your one thought be one of gratitude. Try to replace any negative, destructive thought with one that gives a different message to your brain and ultimately to your body. Initially, you may not even believe the positive thought, but keep trying and change will begin! A new mental path or habit will eventually emerge. The following are some samples of some negative or harmful thoughts and how they might be re-framed.

I can no longer see well enough to read.
I am grateful for auditory books and music.

There are many things I can no longer do.
I have time now to enjoy some quiet activities I never had time for in the past.

I miss my once active social life.
I am thankful that my best friend called today.

I can no longer hike in the mountains.
I am grateful that I can walk.

While re-framing negative thoughts to positive ones can often be mentally challenging, like gymnastics for the brain, a gratitude journal requires very little time and is simple to do. One day per page divided into morning and evening, number 1-5 under each, and you are done! You have a gratitude journal ready to complete!

There have been times that I have literally begun my day with a thank you for being able to breathe, to move, to hear, to smell, to taste, and to see. There is always something to be grateful for in life and in illness! For instance, think about your body. Look at your hands for a full minute while thinking of all they have done for you…the loved ones or pets they have held and comforted, the food prepared, the pages colored, the flowers or tomatoes picked, the notes played, the gifts wrapped and opened with love….then, thank your hands. Do this exercise with your feet, your heart, your eyes…the list is long!

Another simple gratitude practice that has epiphanic potential is the common practice of saying grace during mealtime. Your bowl of oatmeal sits in front of you, and you say a fleeting "Thank you for this food and the hands that prepared it." Does this sound familiar? While this is a good beginning, let's take gratitude further.

Consider prayerfully and gratefully those that grew and harvested the food, the truck driver who transported it, the stock person who placed it on the grocery-store shelf, the person who may have brought it home to you. Going even deeper, think of your oatmeal's beginnings: the sun, the rain, and the earth with its minerals and nutrients. What about the milk, the cow, the bowl, and the spoon? How much further can you expand your awareness of a simple blessing? Try doing this with everything in your life and feel the epiphany happening within you!

If this is difficult for you, choose just one thing for which you are grateful, even it is just for the air that you breathe. If it is all you can pull from within, write it 5 times in the morning. And again, in the evening. Make it your mantra and let it grow!

Can you see the holiness in those things you take for granted– a paved road or a washing machine? If you concentrate on finding what is good in every situation, you will discover that your life will suddenly be filled with gratitude, a feeling that nurtures the soul. Rabbi Harold Kushner

4

Exercise

Those who think they have not time for bodily exercise will sooner or later have to find time for illness. Edward Stanley

For me, exercise is one of my most powerful and favorite healers. Many associate the word "exercise" with drudgery, but I consider it to be moving joyfully with life! From childhood to the present, swimming, horseback riding, ballet, walking, and yoga have been forms of exercise that I have loved. Swimming was not only fun: competitive swimming coupled with ballet yielded a level of fitness that is quite addicting! To this day, I do not feel exactly right unless I exercise every day. Moving, even gently, each morning loosens my joints and muscles, gets my circulation flowing, and provides energy. If my focus, energy, or creativity lags during the day, an exercise break always restores me. Along with loving the way movement makes me feel, being surrounded by beauty, whether I am outdoors, in my favorite room, feeling water flowing softly over my skin, or hearing lovely music as I dance, is the reason that I have continued to exercise throughout my life. If you dislike exercise or are bored while doing it, try something different! If it is painful or makes you feel terrible for days afterward, then what you are doing is not the exercise for you. On the other hand, if your routine makes you smile, brings you a sense of well-being, and you enjoy or even love it, you have discovered the type of exercise that you will continue!

Exercise is truly a magic potion, and if it could be bottled as a medication, most of us would probably rush to purchase it! Countless excuses to avoid exercise are the subjects of many jokes, but if you find something that you truly enjoy, making time for it on a regular basis will be simple. If cost is an issue, there are many types of exercise options that cost very little or may even be free! If you are dealing with chronic illness, the excuse may be that you are unable to exercise or simply don't feel well enough to participate. And those are valid reasons. Before you toss the exercise option in the trash, consider what exercise can do for you:

- relieves stress
- reduces blood pressure, blood sugar, bad cholesterol, and appetite,
- enhances and regulates the immune system
- increases good cholesterol, metabolism, circulation and energy
- improves bone density, muscle strength, and balance
- improves mood and mental clarity
- relaxes muscles
- enhances sleep
- may reduce the risk of Alzheimer's Disease
- may reduce the risk of some cancers

A mixture of aerobic, strengthening, and flexibility exercises should be included in order to reap these benefits, but realistically, having a chronic illness can impose limitations in many cases. First, let's look at the suggested routines for life in a perfect world: life without chronic illness.

It is recommended that aerobic exercise, which includes brisk walking, jogging, swimming, and cycling, be done three times per week for a minimum of 30 minutes each time. The good news is that 10-minute increments throughout the day are also effective! Parking the car at the far end of the parking lot, pulling weeds for 10 minutes, and choosing the stairs instead of the elevator all count. Being stressed generates excess energy, and aerobic activity is a perfect way to dissipate this energy. Even if it is not possible to engage in a strenuous activity when stressed, regular aerobic exercise can drain chronic stress before it becomes a problem!

Strength training can also help with the release of stressful energy and should be done two to three times weekly for 20 to 30 minutes. Light weights, 2 to 5 pounds are best, and if weights are not available, large cans of vegetables or bottled water can be substituted! Along with stress reduction, benefits from strength training include strong muscles that burn calories more efficiently, a reduction in the risk of osteoporosis, a lessening in the pain from arthritis or chronic back issues, and improvement in stamina and balance. Recent studies indicate that strength-building exercise may be the most beneficial exercise for reducing the risk of Alzheimer's Disease.

Another study focused on nursing home residents who had lost their strength and independence. After participating in a simple and gentle weight-lifting program for 10 minutes daily, 3 to 4 times per week, residents regained strength, confidence, and the ability to attend to their activities of daily living. If you find lifting weights for even a short amount of time to be boring, try lifting while watching your favorite 30-minute TV show!

Stretching or flexibility exercises finish this triad. Muscles tend to shorten, weaken, and become stiff with age, making the body prone to injury & stress, and stretching muscles may actually make them stronger! Stretching relaxes tight, tense muscles that often accompany stress and improves your posture and balance! Deep stretches should be included after mild to moderate exercise when muscles are warm, and light stretching, and gentle yoga are excellent to do when muscles are tight from stress or to promote a good night's sleep.

Overall, this is a rigorous schedule to follow, and the chronically ill may be overwhelmed or even give up the idea of exercising after reading these recommendations. Please don't give up! Remember the 10-minute increments throughout the day and the 10 minutes of light weightlifting several times weekly? Those are excellent places to begin. Every chronic condition and every individual are different! Each has different limitations and prognoses. There are usually good days, not-so-good days, and, unfortunately, bad days associated with lengthy illnesses. There may be times when you can do no exercise and times when you may be able to follow the guidelines above. Know your limits, know your body, and work with them!

I do know that since my lupus was diagnosed, there have many times that I wouldn't have left the couch if I hadn't had a ballet class that I was expected to attend. I also know that I felt better afterward! Certainly, if I were experiencing an active flare, I listened. I rested. I nurtured myself. If, however, I was dealing with my usual state of aching muscles and joints and possibly an unrelenting bout of fatigue, I pushed myself out of the door and was glad that I did. You have to know your own body and know it intimately! Are you truly unable to try any exercise today, or might the stiffness, pain, listlessness, and possibly depression respond to some gentle movement? Once you learn to hear your body's message, listen to the message your mind is giving.

From Chapter 2, remember that our thoughts are powerful tools of healing, and our physical, emotional, and spiritual beings listen to all of our thoughts. With that in mind, remember to be equally aware of negative thoughts. A positive thought such as "My energy and pain levels are not good today, but I will do 15 minutes of gentle, restorative stretches for myself" can send messages of healing to your body! The opposing thought "I'm sick of being tired and in pain, and there is no use in doing any exercise today or ever" can be destructive to the mind, body, and spirit!

Two Wolves is a Cherokee Indian legend that describes the power of our beliefs and our thoughts, whether they be good or bad.

An old Cherokee is teaching his grandson about life. "A fight is going on inside me," he said to the boy.
"It is a terrible fight and it is between two wolves. One is evil – he is anger, envy, sorrow, regret, greed, arrogance, self-pity, guilt, resentment, inferiority, lies, false pride, superiority, and ego." He continued, "The other is good – he is joy, peace, love, hope, serenity, humility, kindness, benevolence, empathy, generosity, truth, compassion, and faith. The same fight is going on inside you – and inside every other person, too."
The grandson thought about it for a minute and then asked his grandfather, "Which wolf will win?"
The old Cherokee simply replied, "The one you feed."

This wonderful story is yet another reminder about the power of choosing responses and thoughts! Be careful what you choose to think, what message you send to your body and mind, which wolf you feed! Let your thought be positive and then move whatever you can, whenever you can!

There is exciting news, however, for those who are unable to exercise or who may only be able to participate in limited exercise. Previously, I emphasized the incredible power that thoughts have on the mind, body, and spirit. Even knowing this, I was astounded to learn several years ago the degree to which thoughts can effect change in the body! Various studies have shown that the act of imagining a muscle being exercised increases strength, whether that muscle is at rest in bed or being used during a workout. While active exercise is best, for those whose strength and mobility have been impaired by aging, illness, or stroke, for example, this finding has the potential to change lives!

As I mentioned earlier, exercise has always been part of my life. Early in adulthood, I discovered that if I could exercise for even a short period of time when I first got out of bed, that the day began more smoothly. Not only did I feel better, but I functioned better.

Like so many others, I was a single, working mother with young children, and my days were busy. By getting up a mere 15 or 20 minutes earlier, I had a quiet block of time for my own. Through experimentation, I eventually developed a morning exercise routine that I named my easy 8's. For 8 minutes, I would do a gentle sequence of head-to-toe loosening and stretching movements. Each movement was done to a count of 8. If I had time, I would either repeat them or add 8 minutes of core strengthening.

As the years passed and the health issues began, I found that on most days, regardless of how badly I felt, that the easy 8's were not only doable, but necessary to my well-being! These gentle range of motion movements seemed to loosen my muscles and lubricate my joints. During the good times, I would play with this routine, adding deeper stretching, strength, balance, and even aerobic movements to different styles of music.

My easy 8's then became an important part of my last, and most meaningful, nursing position: parish nursing! Part of my ministry as a parish nurse was to lead an exercise class that I designed for all ages that would focus on promoting balance, strength, and flexibility. The easy 8's evolved into this class that addressed the whole person, and I called it Mind, Body, & Spirit. Done to various classical music, hymns, or chants, Mind, Body, & Spirit begins with a brief prayer or devotion. Using movements from the disciplines of ballet, yoga, and Pilates, it begins with the easy 8's to awaken the body. Next, strengthening work for all muscle groups and whole body stretching complete the movements before ending with a healing meditation, silent relaxation, and a gratitude prayer offered for the gift of exercise and the health and restoration it brings!

If exercise could be packed into a pill, it would be the single most widely prescribed and beneficial medicine in the nation.

Dr. Robert Butler, founder of the National Institute on Aging

The Easy 8's

The Easy 8's are done in a standing position. For support, place your hands on the back of a sturdy chair- or even the kitchen counter!

Begin by being mindful of your posture (tall with shoulders slightly back and down). Tighten the muscles of your thighs and engage your abdomen by pulling your navel toward your spine.

Relax your breathing by inhaling and exhaling <u>slowly</u> through your nose during each movement.

Example: Inhale 2-3-4 then exhale 2-3-4 while doing <u>slow</u> movements to a count of 4.

Begin loosening your joints and muscles and increasing blood flow starting at the top of the head and working down to the toes.

1. Neck - tiny circles in each direction (clockwise to count of 4, counterclockwise to count of 4 while inhaling and exhaling slowly!)
2. Neck - looking over each shoulder to count of 4
3. Neck – tilt right ear toward right shoulder, clasp left wrist and stretch gently, repeat to left
4. Shoulders – circle forward, reverse, rolling shoulders back and squeezing shoulder blades down and together, then shrug (4-count each)
5. Shoulders – intertwine fingers over your head, invert, & stretch toward ceiling
6. Wash windows in a clockwise and counterclockwise direction – repeat with both arms
7. Hands – stretch towards ceiling, clinch, open, keeping thumbs and fingers straight, touch thumb

tip to fingertips, clinch, open again followed by wrist circles

8. Arms out to side, rotate from shoulders palms up, palms down

9. Twist gently at waist

10. Stretch from the waist laterally to right without leaning forward, bringing left arm up and across the head, repeat to other side

11. Hips – stand with R leg raised in marching position, make circles to both directions, repeat with L leg

12. Gently swing each leg forward and backward from the hips

13. R foot – point to the side, flex, repeat, then draw circles with the right big toe, repeat with L foot

14. With feet facing forward, press gently against the toes of the right foot, feeling toes spread apart, repeat with left foot

15. With feet rotated out at 11:00 and 1:00 o'clock, Bend both knees, and keeping upper body erect and knees over the feet, lower 4 times with each time lowering a little further. As you do this exercise, imagine that your back is pressed against a wall and that it slides down the wall as the knees bend. This keeps you from leaning forward

16. Feet & calves – rise to balls of feet, come down slowly. Repeat 8 times. Balance on last one

17. Stretch calves - with both feet facing forward, place right foot 2-3 feet behind you, and keeping both feet flat on floor, press toward bent left foot with left knee bent. Right leg should remain straight. Repeat with left foot behind

18. Balance, stretch & strengthen — Place feet wide apart, with toes angled out at approximately 10 and 2 o'clock. Breathe in (arms and upper body stretch up with legs straight), breathe out (arms come to prayer position as legs bend), squeeze inner thighs as you straighten your legs, press hands engaging arm muscles while in prayer position

19. Stretch from the hips forward, keeping the back straight as you go forward. Pull your navel to your spine and roll up one vertebra at a time to return to standing straight

20. End standing sequence with a spinal stretch. Stand as described in the beginning. Stretch arms and entire body toward the ceiling (on tiptoe if you can balance), then fold down on yourself with knees bent, chest comes towards thighs, chin to chest, arms bend, and elbows swing behind. Slowly unfold by beginning to straighten knees, straightening arms as chest lifts. Now you are back to your upright standing position with your chin tilted slightly upward.

During these standing exercises, try to keep your navel firmly against your spine, and your upper thighs, inner thighs, and glutes (or buttocks) firm and engaged. You will be strengthening your abdomen, lower back, legs, and hips! When tightening the abdomen, make sure you leave space to breathe fully!

Always check with your healthcare provider before beginning any exercise program!

5

Sleep

Sleep is the golden chain that ties health and our bodies together. Thomas Dekker

Jason Bourne, in the series of books called <u>The Bourne Trilogy</u> by Robert Ludlum, states that sleep is a weapon, and if you have chronic illness, it is a weapon that you desperately need! Bourne knows that in order to survive, he must rest, and he always sleeps before confronting an enemy. While you may not be facing enemies on a daily basis, how many stressors, conflicts, health issues or personal crises do you encounter? Without adequate sleep, you quickly begin to notice difficulty concentrating, impaired reaction time, irritability, memory impairment, and difficulty staying awake during important situations – like driving on the interstate or even an important meeting! As sleep deprivation becomes chronic, you may also experience a poorly functioning immune system. Severe sleep deprivation can sometimes result in disorientation and hallucinations! Sleep is critical in reducing stress. Almost all chronically stressed people are fatigued, and people who are tired don't handle stressful situations very well. The Mayo Clinic cites studies that suggest that sleep loss (less than 7 hours per night) may have wide-ranging effects on the cardiovascular, endocrine, immune, and nervous systems, including the following:

- Obesity in adults and children

- Diabetes and impaired glucose tolerance
- Cardiovascular disease and hypertension
- Anxiety symptoms
- Depressed mood
- Alcohol use

Most adults need 7 to 9 hours of sleep per night. If you are in good health, there are two easy ways to know if you are getting enough sleep: if you wake refreshed without the need of an alarm clock and if you have good energy during the day! Having a chronic illness, however, changes the picture. First of all, you may actually need more sleep, and secondly, a chronic illness may make it more difficult to get the quantity and quality of sleep that your body needs. There are many reasons that chronic illness can disrupt your night-time sleep cycle.

- Pain
- Sleeping during the day because of fatigue
- Anxiety or depression
- Worry or stress
- Medications such as prednisone that are stimulating
- Medications that are sedating can actually disrupt normal sleep. Some medications for sleep, pain, anxiety, and depression may be in the sedating category.

Although sleep doesn't seem to get as much attention as nutrition and exercise, most healthcare practitioners agree that sleep is a powerful healer, or as Bourne might say, a powerful weapon against disease! Sleep is when the body restores and repairs itself. While the following simple and free suggestions apply to everyone, not everyone can adhere to all of them. Hopefully, you can find some ideas for making changes that will improve your sleep. Your health will appreciate it! I know from experience that I can count on this fact: whether I am having a flare or am in remission, the following day is a struggle if I don't sleep well!

- Try to go to sleep and get up at the same time every day. This will put your body into a good "sleep-wake rhythm."
- Caffeine, nicotine, and heavy or spicy meals close to bedtime may make it difficult to fall asleep.
- Try having your last caffeinated drink or chocolate at lunch or even earlier in the day.
- Alcohol interferes with the ability to sleep deeply.
- Regular exercise is helpful. Strenuous exercise is best earlier in the day and gentle yoga or stretching may be relaxing closer to bedtime. The easy 8's are perfect for evening as well!
- Decrease fluids right before bed so that a full bladder doesn't awaken you
- Have a good sleep environment: comfortable bed, cool temperature, and as dark as possible.
- Don't use your bedroom as an office or TV room. Let your body and brain know that the bed is associated with sleeping.
- A warm (not hot) bath just before bedtime.
- Prayer, meditation, and relaxation techniques (see Chapter 6) relieve anxiety and reduce muscle tension.
- Avoid stimulating or stressful reading materials, TV programs, or discussions
- If you don't fall asleep within 15 to 30 minutes, get up, go into another room and read or watch TV until sleepy.

If you still have insomnia or poor sleep quality, you may want to try the following treatments or the Complementary Alternative Medicine treatments listed below.

- Cognitive Behavioral Therapy (CBT), biofeedback, or hypnotherapy sessions with a licensed therapist or counselor
- Natural remedies include herbs such as chamomile tea, valerian, and lemon balm and supplements such as melatonin. Combinations of these and other ingredients may also be found in health food stores and drug stores.
- Aromatherapy with essential oils like lavender
- Acupuncture and massage
- Yoga and gentle stretching
- Music therapy

When considering herbs or supplements, always check with your healthcare providers first. Some may have side effects or interact with your current medications. With some medical conditions, certain herbs and supplements may be harmful. Always purchase these products from a reputable retailer in order to get a safe, quality product!

After years of trial and error, I have discovered that what works best for me is to keep a regular schedule, avoid caffeine after lunch, avoid stressful TV near bedtime, gentle stretching, and 3-5 mg of melatonin. A cool, comfortable bedroom also helps, but the others are mandatory for me! It also can't hurt (and you may resent me for mentioning this one) that my dear, supportive husband gently rubs my neck and upper back each night when I go to bed. Back to gratitude...he's at the top of my list! May your sleep be healing, and may your dreams be sweet!

And if tonight my soul may find her peace in sleep, and sink in good oblivion, and in the morning wake like a new opened flower then I have been dipped again in God, and new created.
D.H. Lawrence

6

Stress and Relaxation

It's not stress that kills us, it is our reaction to it. Hans Selye

Life is filled with stress. Sometimes stress is useful, such as when we see a car approaching in your lane, and the stress reaction enables you to avoid it. Other times it is not. For instance, you may have a job that you dislike or an illness that you can't manage. The bad kind of stress can occur when you feel you have no choices open to you. Good stressors include a new marriage, the birth of a child, and even Christmas, while divorce, accidents or a death in the family create bad stress. Any type of change causes stress, and as long as you are alive, you just can't avoid it! By learning to recognize and manage stress, you can protect yourself from the potential harm that it can cause.

In order to understand the stress response, you need to learn what happens inside you when you are faced with a stressor. It is very complicated, but in a nutshell, the brain receives the message that there is a threat or a change and alerts the rest of your body. Surprisingly, your body can't differentiate between good stress and bad stress: it simply reacts! Glands send chemicals like adrenalin into the bloodstream to ready you for either "fight or flight." Heart rate and blood pressure rise, blood flow increases in the muscles, and blood sugar and fats in the blood increase so that extra fuel is available. Cortisol, from the adrenal gland, rushes into your bloodstream to prevent loss of fluids and to thicken the blood in case of possible wounds. It also causes the immune system to stop its valuable work and inflammation to decrease. All energy is re-routed in order to deal with the perceived threat—the stressor.

Once upon a time, these responses enabled your distant ancestors to survive threats from wild animals and hostile clans, but today this response can cause damage to your body when it happens regularly throughout each day. More damage occurs when stress becomes chronic, and if your stress level lasts for long periods of time, serious and sometimes permanent conditions may occur.

Chronic elevated levels of cortisol and other stress response hormones can cause diabetes or insulin resistance, heart disease, underactive or overactive immune system, obesity, high cholesterol, liver disease, and osteoporosis. Some believe that cancer may be triggered by stress.

Emotionally, chronic stress can cause sleep disorders, eating issues, anxiety, and depression. If stressed, you may also notice appetite changes, insomnia, frequent colds or other illnesses, irritability, fatigue, poor concentration, and feeling like you want to withdraw from your family or friends. Some even turn to substance abuse to try to relieve the symptoms. There are many self-help books and audio and video products that can help you learn about stress management practices. If after trying relaxation and some of the following ways to manage your stress you find that you are still having stress-related problems, please talk with your doctor, minister, or licensed counselor!

Ways to Manage Stress

- Relaxation strategies that can slow the pulse, decrease blood pressure, and relax muscles include meditation, Tai Chi, yoga, progressive muscle relaxation, and visualization.
- Exercise: again, the easy 8's are perfect for calming the body.
- Good Nutrition
- Relationships/Family/Friends
- Hobbies/Recreation
- Sleep/Rest
- Laughter
- Prayer/Spirituality - Francis de Sales wrote: "Every one of us needs half an hour of prayer each day, except when we are busy – then we need an hour."

Wayne Muller wrote a book called <u>Sabbath,</u> in which he talks about the importance of making time for the Sabbath. Whether it's a minute, an hour, or a day, this time is critical for our wellbeing. This time is for renewal and for protection from the busyness and the stressors of modern life. He goes on to say that if you don't make time for the Sabbath, your illness will become your Sabbath. In illness, especially a serious illness, you are forced to rest and let go of demands and expectations. He gives a powerful example of how mindfulness and breath work to create Sabbath times during the day:

In the Buddhist community of Plum Village, Thich Nhat Hanh, a Vietnamese monk periodically rings a Mindfulness Bell. Upon hearing the bell, everyone stops, and takes three silent, mindful breaths. Then they are free to continue their work, awakened ever so slightly by the Sabbath pause of mindfulness. We can choose anything to stop us like this – the telephone ringing, a stoplight when we are driving, whenever our hand touches a doorknob, before we eat or drink. Choose one common act during your day to serve as a Sabbath pause. Whenever this arises – whenever you touch a doorknob or hear the telephone – simply stop, take three silent, mindful breaths, and then go through the door or answer the phone.

Even such small changes can calm the mind, body, and spirit thus reducing the stress response, and an even more powerful stress-reducer is doing your breath work for 5 minutes twice a day.

Sit up tall and straight, or lie in a comfortable position, preferably on your back. Imagine that your lungs are empty, flat balloons! Breathe deeply to a count of 5 into the bottom of your balloons and pause for a moment. Your abdomen and ribcage will gently expand. Your chest barely moves. Your abdomen and ribcage begin to sink as the air pushed gently from the bottom of your balloons as you exhale to a count of 5. Pause for a moment and begin the cycle again. Focus on the counted breath. If unwanted thoughts come to the surface, simply let them float by. Trying to force yourself to not think only gives these thoughts more power. This will probably take some practice initially, but soon you will notice a new sense of calmness and focus that not only lasts for several hours but becomes a part of you!

Over the years, I have found many ways that help me manage stress. Individually or in combination, I have experimented with finding whatever works for me at a particular time in my life, and the ones that have been most helpful follow in no particular order

• Exercise: Ballet, yoga, swimming, and gardening are just some examples. Strenuous exercise or housework can help an anxious or even agitated stress reaction to almost evaporate, while a gentler form of movement can relieve muscle tension and worry.

• Prayer, breath work, or meditation: These disciplines help calm and focus a busy mind.

• Aromatherapy: Essential oils, like lavender, are soothing, especially when dispersed in a mister over a period of hours.

• Music: Some music is calming, and some is fun or energizing. The choice is important — it depends on the mood!

• Limiting my exposure to negativity: I watch the news twice daily. Five minutes of national news, five minutes of local, and a few minutes of sports and weather in the morning and evening is enough to keep me informed. To me, social media should be social, and I limit my time there as well. I love to celebrate friends' birthdays, see pictures of their grandchildren, share their joys, and support them in times of sorrow. It can become a stealer of precious time and a major stressor when anger, resentments, and arguments replace the social aspect.

> *... As healing energy and affirmations*
> *embrace my very cells,*
> *The dance begins, I am whole,*
> *And I pray through pliés...*

I have found that the way I begin my day often sets the tone for all that follows. If I can manage my stress before it begins, it loses its power over me. I arise early. This is my time. My Sabbath time, as Muller would say. I put on some soft, beautiful music, take a deep, cleansing breath, and begin my easy 8's, the movement routine mentioned in Chapter 4, to gently awaken my body. These are followed by doing some stretches on the floor, and then I begin my morning prayers and blessings. I may give thanks for the day, my body, for music. I ask for blessings of well-being, peace, and an awareness of God's constant love for all those that I love. Without moving from this place of prayer, I breathe. I meditate. I listen. The music continues during breakfast. While eating, I read. I read only what is inspirational or simply beautiful during this time, and I have learned about and traveled to some amazing places without leaving my table. As the day goes on, I try to be mindful about my gratitude practice.

Thank you for this food, for those who grew it, who packaged it, and for my husband who brought it home for me.
Thank you for the sunlight that streams through so many windows and the rainbows dancing across the wall created by the prisms that my mother gave me.
Thank you for this cat who makes me laugh and for family and friends.
Thank you for water for showering, drinking, and cleaning my clothes and dishes.

The list is endless if I am truly mindful. My coat of armor in place, I am prepared to manage whatever stress comes my way. I am ready to calmly live my day.

This is another day, O Lord. I know not what it will bring forth, but make me ready, Lord, for whatever it may be. If I am to stand up, help me to stand bravely. If I am to sit still, help me to sit quietly. If I am to lie low, help me to do it patiently. And if I am to do nothing, let me do it gallantly. Make these words more than words, and give me the Spirit of Jesus. Amen.

--The Episcopal Book of Common Prayer

7

Nutrition

The food you eat can be either the safest and most powerful form
of medicine or the slowest form of poison.
Ann Wigmore

Let me begin by saying that since birth, or at least as far
back as I can remember, I have had a love affair with sugar.
Some of my earliest memories involve the cakes my aunt
would make from scratch, or more accurately, licking the
bowls that held the batter. I still lick bowls and have been
known to make a cake solely for the enjoyment of eating the
batter. White flour that is high in gluten for tenderness, milk,
real butter, eggs, and white sugar: could it be any
unhealthier? Especially raw?

Yes, I realize that I may someday die from salmonella
from eating raw eggs, but addictions are powerful, and I
rationalize that at least I will die with cake batter on my lips!
After all, I try to eat only cake made from scratch —
preservatives and artificial ingredients are simply toxic!
Brownies, cookies, cobbler, doughnuts. I love them all, but
cake — and its batter — is my absolute favorite. I will go so far
to say that it feeds my soul, and that is important!

So, in all honesty, for most of my life my eating habits
have not been particularly healthy. I was fortunate in that I
never have had a very large appetite. Combining that with
the fact that I was an extremely picky eater during childhood
and young adulthood led me to the one habit I had going in
my favor: my style of eating. I have never been one to
overeat, but I also have never missed a meal! Breakfast,
lunch, and dinner with a small snack in the

afternoon has always been a comfortable routine for me, because I do not like to be hungry nor do I enjoy feeling stuffed. My weight has been relatively the same since my mid-teens. Most of my activities involved wearing either a dance leotard or a competitive-style swimsuit. Not only was I instantly aware of weight gain, but ballet pointe shoes are not forgiving of extra pounds carried on one's toes! From adulthood forward, I have never paid much attention to weight or checking calories on labels. The discipline was quite simple: if my clothes felt snug, I slightly reduced my food intake for several days.

This has always worked well for me, and my joints seem to appreciate the effort. However, by not counting calories, I also neglected something very important. I did not read the food labels. For many years, even decades, I simply wasn't interested.

As lupus flares increased in both frequency and intensity as I reached my forties, I began to pay a little closer attention to my diet. I tried to include at least one green vegetable daily that wasn't a small piece of lettuce on a sandwich, several servings of calcium-rich foods, some fresh fruit, and several servings of whole grains. On most days, I managed to limit my desserts to one per day!

By now I had discovered alternative and natural medicine and found their philosophies fascinating. Some of them complemented my nursing approach and theories of healing. After thorough researching, I began using supplements such as antioxidants, multi-vitamins, and calcium. They sounded as if they might benefit me, and I felt secure in my now "healthy" diet boosted by these supplements.

The flares continued, however, and a chemotherapy medication, methotrexate, was suggested by my MD. A friend, who also happened to be a nurse, suggested that I try homeopathic treatment combined with energy medicine first. Although I was beginning to be quite familiar with alternative treatments, I was skeptical. The homeopathic practitioner did a lengthy evaluation, prescribed a remedy and several supplements, and restricted all dairy, wheat, sugar, and caffeine from my diet. Within weeks, I felt better than I had in many years, my energy was great, and my lab work had improved to almost normal levels.

For six months, I remained on this treatment regimen and enjoyed the well-being that accompanied it. Thanksgiving, Christmas, and several birthday parties later, I gave in to temptation and gradually began to include the restricted foods into my meals. I still remember the first time I ate dairy and the nausea that quickly followed. And the first dessert with wheat and sugar. The resulting headache was vicious! I also remember thinking, "Wow, that's a really strong message!"

I ignored the message, however, and the autoimmune symptoms began to creep back. My fifties came, and with the exception of flares occurring every two to three years, I felt fairly good. Chronic mild fatigue along with muscle and joint pain were the norm that I adapted to, and except for adding several salads a week — always with fat-laden buttermilk dressing that probably did more harm than good — to my prior diet plan, little changed in my eating habits.

Just before my 60th birthday, however, something did change. The autoimmune response seemed to gather speed and strength and the resulting inflammation was very difficult to manage. The next few years involved multiple doctor visits, medication changes, absences from work, periods of being unable to dance, and what I now recognize as mild depression. When I wasn't working, I was in my pajamas. I was not well, and I was not enjoying my life.

I woke up one morning in early March of 2013, and I thought, "I am done with this. I cannot control this disease, but there is one thing that I can control. I can control what I put in my mouth, and if it's not good fuel, full of nutrients, and healing, it won't enter this body!" Dietary changes had helped me once before, and I believed they could do it again. The questions I would ask before swallowing anything were:

- Is this food a good fuel?
- Does it have good nutritional value?
- Is it healing?

If the answers were no, I didn't eat it. These three criteria became my new guidelines, and I was relentless in adhering to them. This new philosophy of eating and nutrition led me to the anti-inflammatory diet. This diet has been described by and recommended by various healthcare practitioners including the Sjogren's Syndrome Foundation and the Harvard Women's Health Watch. Chronic inflammation, even at low levels, has been linked to a variety of serious, chronic illnesses. Studies have shown that an anti-inflammatory diet is effective in reducing inflammation while enhancing health. Along with reducing the production of inflammatory chemicals, the anti-inflammatory diet also addresses which foods and products to avoid that have the potential to actually increase inflammation.

Similar to the Mediterranean Diet, which is high in fruits, vegetables, nuts, whole grains, fish, and healthy oils, the anti-inflammatory diet focuses on whole foods that are rich in nutrients.

Anti-inflammatory foods

- Colorful fruits and vegetables, such as spinach, kale, sweet potatoes, beets, carrots, berries, cherries, oranges, tomatoes
- Healthy fats, including omega 3 oils found in extra virgin olive oil, raw nuts, seeds, ground flax seed, avocados, fatty fish (salmon, mackerel, sardines)
- Healthy proteins, including small amounts of lean, organic meat like grass-fed beef, free-range chicken, eggs from free-range chicken
- Grains, including brown rice, whole-wheat, oats, barley, quinoa, amaranth
- Spices such as ginger, turmeric, garlic, oregano, and cinnamon, and pepper
- Tea (brewed green or black)
-

Inflammatory foods to avoid

- Trans, saturated, or hydrogenated fats, margarine, shortening, lard
- High fructose corn syrup
- Sugar and hidden sugars that end with the letters "ose" or "ol" such as fructose, sucrose, mannitol, sorbitol
- Most processed or refined foods that have added sugars, preservatives, and refined carbohydrates. These include pastries, most cereals, white flour, white rice, white potatoes, sugar, breads and red meat.

The following suggestions are simple ways to remember my criteria and these anti-inflammatory diet guidelines:

- Shop the perimeter of the grocery store where you will find fresh, colorful produce and foods.
- Try to "eat the rainbow" with your produce each day. Different colors of fruits and vegetables have different vitamins, minerals, and other nutrients.
- Always read the labels and be wary of too many ingredients or ingredients that you either can't pronounce or have no idea what they are!

This is the style of eating that matched my 3 criteria, and I began to proudly declare that kale had become my new best friend! I do admit that I ate a piece of cake—homemade, of course—for my grandson's birthday, but I can honestly say that I had not missed the sugar. The triad of good fuel, nutrient dense, and healing qualities brought me once again to a new level of energy within the first 2 months and to remarkable lab values within 6 months. I was in control. Lupus and Sjogren's can never be cured, but I now knew the dietary formula that my body needed to keep them happy and in remission.

The doctor of the future will no longer treat the human frame with drugs, but rather will cure and prevent disease with nutrition. Thomas Edison

8

Neurotoxicity & the Nervous System

The body is a sacred garment. It's your first and last garment; it is what you enter life in and what you depart life with, and it should be treated with honor. Martha Graham

In order to understand the rest of my journey, reading this brief chapter is important! Having just a basic understanding of neurons and the nervous system will help in understanding neurotoxicity and its effect on the nervous system.

Neurons, or nerve cells are the body's messengers. The body has billions of neurons, more than the stars in the Milky Way! Most estimates are that there are about 100 billion neurons in the brain and around 13.5 million in the spinal cord.

Neurons have specialized functions, and the nervous system, made up of these neurons, is the body's inner communication system! The nerve cells take in information, and the brain then interprets this information in order to understand what's going on both outside and inside the body. This allows a person to respond to and interact with his or her surrounding environment and to control body functions.

The nervous system and its billions of neurons are divided into two parts based on their location in the body:

the central nervous system and the peripheral nervous system. The central nervous system consists of the brain and spinal cord. It receives information from the peripheral nervous system, analyzes it, and coordinates the activity of the entire nervous system. The peripheral nervous system includes all peripheral nerves, the nerves that are outside of the brain and spinal cord. It can coordinate everything from bending the knee to regulating blood pressure.

The central nervous system and the peripheral nervous system are further divided into the voluntary and involuntary nervous systems. The body's voluntary nervous system controls things a person is aware of and can control consciously, such as moving their head, arms, legs, or other body parts. Also called the autonomic nervous system, the involuntary system controls processes in the body that a person doesn't consciously control. The autonomic nervous system is always active, and among other critical body processes, regulates a person's heart rate, blood pressure, breathing, and metabolism.

The autonomic part of the peripheral nervous system is divided once again into the enteric, sympathetic, and parasympathetic systems. The sympathetic nervous system, our fight or flight system, tells the body to get ready! Whether it's a bear, an impending accident, a job interview, or unusual or stressful physical or mental activity, the system puts us in high gear! Refer to Chapter 6 on Stress and Relaxation if needed for a review about what happens when this system activates.

The parasympathetic nervous system restores the body; it brings the body back to a calm and relaxed state.

The enteric nervous system is often referred to as the second brain! It communicates with the sympathetic and parasympathetic nervous system but is also able to function independently. Beginning in the upper part of the esophagus, it covers the entire gastrointestinal tract and communicates primarily through the vagus nerve. Vagus means "wandering" in Latin, and this large, multi-branched nerve functions as commander of the parasympathetic nervous system. Its fibers touch the tongue, throat, vocal cords, lungs, heart, stomach, intestines, and glands that produce anti-stress chemicals and hormones.

If your eyes are glazing over or if you're yawning or even asleep by now, you have met your parasympathetic nervous system! I realize that this all sounds very complicated, and that's because it is! The nervous system is a miraculous communication network, and each neuron has a specific role. Every organ, every muscle, every cell, and even every thought is dependent on a neuron receiving a message and firing its response correctly and consistently.

What happens to this complex system when a neurotoxic event occurs? The National Institute of Neurological Disorders and Stroke describes neurotoxicity as an exposure to natural or manmade toxic substances (neurotoxins) that alters the normal activity of the nervous system. This can eventually disrupt or even kill neurons, key cells that transmit and process signals in the brain and other parts of the nervous system. Neurotoxicity can result from exposure to substances used in chemotherapy, radiation treatment, prescription drug therapies, and organ transplants, as well as exposure to heavy metals such as lead and mercury, certain foods and food additives, pesticides, industrial and/or cleaning solvents, cosmetics, and some naturally occurring substances. Some of the symptoms resulting from cell death include autonomic nervous system dysfunction, weakness, headaches, loss of motor or movement control, and deterioration in the ability to perceive, think, problem-solve, and learn. These symptoms may appear immediately after exposure or be delayed. The prognosis depends upon the length and degree of exposure and the severity of neurological injury. In some instances, neurotoxicity can be fatal. In others, patients may survive but not fully recover. In others, Individuals may recover completely. It has also been found to be a major risk factor for development of neuro-degenerative diseases such as Alzheimer's disease .

It's now time to apply this detailed and possibly confusing information that you have just read! Take a few minutes and picture a 24-hour period in your life. Think of everything that you and your body does from the time you awaken to the time you fall asleep and then awaken again. Imagine the billions of neurons working perfectly and continuously in order to make those 24 hours possible. Finally, imagine a neurotoxin entering your body, like a heat-seeking missile. Neurons are its target. Billions of neurons with specific missions that are the body's entire communication system. Some neurons may be unaffected, and some may be severely damaged and may regenerate weeks, months, or years later. Some may even die. The communication network is broken, and the 24-hour period that you pictured earlier may not be possible again. In June of 2015, a neurotoxin entered my body and my life, and the heat-seeking missile was Levaquin.

The leafless trees, with their black branches stretched hysterically in every direction, looked to him like illustrations of a central nervous system racked by disease: studies of human suffering anatomized against the winter sky.
Edward St. Aubyn, Dunbar

9

Levaquin

When you reach the end of your light and step out into the darkness, faith is knowing that your feet will land on solid ground or that you will be taught to fly.
Edward Teller (paraphrased)

Prayers of gratitude, positive thinking, exercise, sleep, stress management, and diet were the core of the self-prescribed healthcare plan that had evolved over many years. The anti-inflammatory diet was the last piece of the puzzle, so to speak, and I was confident that future flares would be mild and less frequent. Throughout the remainder of 2013 and for most of 2014, the autoimmune diseases responded well. In December of 2014, I experienced an unrelenting flare. Joint and muscle pain along with sporadic bouts of fever kept me barely functional. I was encouraged to work from home one day per week and made calls and wrote notes while curled on the couch in my pajamas. I dressed for Christmas Day but remember nothing else about that time with my family. I was eventually placed on methotrexate, a chemotherapy medication to suppress and calm my immune system. This flare gradually subsided over a period of months, but I remained on methotrexate. Knowing that my immune response was suppressed, or as my doctor described it, "chemically disabled," I was very careful about avoiding exposure to contagious diseases.

Fate and a large dose of bad luck must have conspired to initiate my greatest health challenge to this point. On Friday evening, June the 12th, I became ill with a high fever and cough. On the next day, Saturday, June the 13th, I was seen at an urgent care clinic and diagnosed with pneumonia. A fluoroquinolone antibiotic called Levaquin was prescribed, and the unimaginable began.

Although I have had lupus and Sjögren's Syndrome for decades, I made a choice early on to not let these autoimmune disorders define me. Instead, I had chosen to be grateful to this pair for making me appreciate each day. I had chosen to pursue the things "now" that brought joy and meaning instead of waiting for "someday." I had raised a family, been a swim team coach, a piano teacher, a Licensed Professional Counselor, and enjoyed a nursing career that spanned over 30 years in a variety of settings that included hospital, community mental health, correctional, hospice, and parish nursing.

I had retired from the state of NC in 2006, and at the time that I developed pneumonia, I was employed full-time as a Parish Nurse at First Presbyterian Church in Morganton, NC. I loved being a Parish Nurse. It was the most rewarding vocation imaginable. My 10-year anniversary was around the corner, and I hoped to remain in this ministry for many years to come.

I was extremely health conscious, and I was very active: I exercised daily; had studied ballet since 1955 and still performed; I once swam in the Junior Olympics and continued fitness swimming; I lifted weights 2-3 times per week; and I led the weekly exercise class mentioned in Chapter 4 that consisted of ballet, yoga, and Pilates movements. My husband and I loved visiting our National Parks, and we walked together regularly in order to be able to hike when we traveled.

This is who I was before June of 2015. This is who I was before Levaquin. When I was prescribed a 10-day course of Levaquin on June the 13th, I already knew about the risk of tendon rupture and was warned about strenuous exercise. Other side effects were not discussed with me, and my focus was solely on getting well. As a healthcare provider myself, I trusted the treatment plan prescribed.

My biggest concern at this point was that I was depleting my vacation days that I had saved for an upcoming trip. My husband and I were to leave in mid-August for a 3-week trip to Yellowstone and the Tetons that would end in Amarillo, Texas for my husband's 50th high-school reunion. We had briefly visited Yellowstone and the Tetons once before and could hardly wait to spend more time in those parks! I finished the Levaquin on June the 22nd. The pneumonia was resolving, and I planned to return to work on the 29th. Our trip was still possible!

The morning of June the 24th began like any other, but if I had known what the next hour, weeks, months, and years would bring, I would have put on my pointe shoes and danced. I would have run…I would have played the piano and worked on stained glass. But we never know what any day will bring. We never know when the things we take for granted might disappear.

While eating breakfast, I thought my hands had gone to sleep. I noticed tingling and prickling, or paresthesia, in both hands. Within one hour, everything I touched—my clothes, a towel—felt like I was grasping a cactus. I saw my internist on June the 25th, and he diagnosed me with peripheral neuropathy due to a probable neurotoxic reaction to Levaquin. Then he said that it might be irreversible! Shocked, I didn't really believe him, but a trickle of fear still washed over me. How could this happen? How could a nurse not know about this possible side effect? Why was I not warned and given a choice? I now know that because I was over age 60, had an autoimmune disease, and was on a steroid and methotrexate, I should not have been prescribed a fluoroquinolone antibiotic. In all fairness, my immune system may not have dealt with the pneumonia effectively due to being suppressed by medication, and the urgent care physician probably thought that I required a strong antibiotic. I also know how my body can be a little strange and often reacts in unusual ways. If I had been informed about the possible adverse reactions to this class of antibiotics, I would not have taken it!

My doctor also told me that if the symptoms worsened, I needed to be seen right away by either him or in the emergency room if his office was closed. Still not believing that this bizarre reaction would not leave as quickly as it had come, I drove home. Armed with extra B12 injections, B-complex supplements, and magnesium that my doctor had recommended to support my nervous system, I thought, "You've got this, you're going to be fine!"

That evening, as I was carrying my humidifier, it suddenly landed in the floor. As water ran in all directions, I realized that the muscles in my arms had simply become limp and let go of the filled container. What just happened here? My arms quickly returned to normal, so I tried to put it out of my mind because there seemed to be no logical explanation.

Several hours later, I noticed an uncomfortable sensation in my feet. Wearing my usual around-the house-fuzzy socks, I thought that I had somehow gotten cat litter or little pebbles inside them. I shook them out and put them back on my feet. The gritty feeling was still there! I changed my socks twice before realization dawned: my feet were now affected.

By the next day, it felt as if I were walking on broken seashells, and the tingling and numbness, the paresthesia, now involved my back, abdomen, chest, feet, and legs. My abdominal muscles and diaphragm were not functioning properly. Even with effort, I could not cough effectively. My shallow cough hardly cleared my throat.

On June the 26th, I developed severe ataxia, or uncontrolled, spastic movements in my legs and arms, severe muscle weakness, and dysphagia, meaning that I choked on almost everything that I ate and drank. I was too weak to stand in the shower, and the one time I attempted a tub bath, I thought that I would drown. I had difficulty remaining in an upright seated position because the muscles in my neck, shoulders, upper back, and core were too weak to support my upper body and head. As my head and upper body began to tilt steadily toward the water, I used all the strength I had in my arms to pull myself over the side of the bathtub. My husband never knew this until much later. I desperately tried to hide this progressive deterioration so as not to worry him. Did I tell my family? My friends? No. They knew I was recovering from the pneumonia and that the antibiotic was causing some odd sensations in my hands and feet. They also knew that I rested or slept— a lot. My thought processes and my judgement were obviously deteriorating as well.

By Sunday, June the 28th, the paresthesia, ataxia, and muscle weakness were markedly worse. I began dropping things. Alone in the house, I had to try once more to do the things people do every day. Perhaps it wasn't as bad as I thought. I had to try.

I could not open a simple drawer: I would reach for the knob, but the spasticity of my movements required me to hold both hands together in order to clasp the knob. Finally, a small success! It was short-lived, though, because I didn't have the strength to pull the drawer open. Then, I fell.

In desperation, to try to make my body move normally and to prove to myself that I was ok, I attempted to wash a load of clothes. I could not open the container of detergent. I then tried my ballet barre exercise routine. The simple ballet movements that I attempted resembled someone having a seizure. I could not force my muscles to respond to the commands that I was giving them. I could not force my diaphragm to take a deep breath or to force a cough from my lungs. Never had I experienced such a sense of defenselessness and no small degree of terror. I fell—again— and sat on the floor and cried.

By now, my diet consisted of liquid nutritional supplements. Even soft foods, if I was able to get them down at all without choking, would simply not move beyond the upper part of my chest.

Denial, that initial refusal to believe that this was truly happening, was now replaced by panic with the realization that I could hardly take care of myself. And it appeared to be getting worse.

I was 64 and had been anxiously waiting to turn 65 for some time. My mother died at age 64, and we shared a similar medical history. Irrationally, I wanted to be past this milestone of sorts and didn't like the way this was developing.

Rationally, I should have called my doctor again by now, and I should have gone to the emergency room. I was not thinking very clearly at this point. I was not only too exhausted to tolerate the long wait that one usually faces in the ER, but I was afraid that I would be exposed to some other contagious disease.

I waited until Monday morning, June the 29th, to see my internist again. Unable to walk without assistance, my husband took me and practically had to carry me. By this time, my breathing had become very shallow, and I was short of breath. My blood pressure was erratic. My doctor admitted me to the hospital, and my hospital record said that I was admitted to Catawba Valley Medical Center with impending respiratory failure due to a neurotoxic reaction to Levaquin. As the heart monitor pads were placed on my chest, I could see the dawning panic in my husband's eyes. He told me later that he felt confident that I would be detoxed from this drug, that some miraculous treatment would remove all traces of toxicity from my body. He was sure that I would return home, perhaps a little fatigued, but in the same condition prior to Levaquin. We had no idea that the damage had been done before I even experienced my first symptom.

Throughout my stay, I required assistance to stand and to do self-care. I had difficulty bringing a cup to my mouth because of extreme weakness and inability to control my arms. Even in these circumstances, denial, desperation, and just plain stubbornness were fierce. Once, while my husband was supporting me to stand beside the bed, I faced him and placed my hands on his shoulders. With his hands around my waist, I worked my feet into ballet first position and began to do relevés, or calf raises. The physical therapist arrived at that moment to do her initial evaluation. "What are you doing?" she asked. "Ballet," I said. When asked why, I responded that the dancer in me had to prove to myself that I could. The nurse in me then added that I was trying to prevent blood clots.

"Wow, you are going to be an interesting patient," she said. "You must understand that even with hard work, recovery could take months, or years." I didn't believe her, and neither did my daughter, who replied without hesitation, "No, you don't understand. My mom has always beaten the odds: she is a hot mess!" Physical therapy began shortly after and consisted of transferring to a wheelchair, limited standing, and attempting several steps with support before needing to rest again.

My breathing remained shallow and the ability to cough effectively continued to be impaired. I also began to experience painful muscle spasms in my neck and back.

One night was particularly bad. Medication brought no relief, and I used the side rails to turn myself over and work myself onto my hands and knees in the bed. My hope was that I could attempt to find some relief from the unrelenting pain by doing the yoga cat and cow positions. While unsuccessful, I suppose the miracle was that I didn't fall out of bed, and I was quite grateful that the physical therapist didn't walk in at that moment!

I was initially on clear liquids. I felt like a hummingbird as my healthy, no-sugar diet of the preceding years was abandoned in the quest for high-calorie, high-protein liquid supplements. A barium swallow study indicated that the nerves leading to my esophagus were damaged. Because of that, the peristalsis, or contractions, in my esophagus was too weak to move solid foods.

Every movement was difficult, agonizing, and exhausting. The consensus between my internist, the hospitalist, the rheumatologist, two neurologists, and the physical therapist was that I had had a severe reaction to the Levaquin that had affected sensory, motor, and autonomic nerve cells— essentially my entire neuromuscular system.

On the 3rd day of hospitalization, as I lay in the bed trying to understand what was happening to me, trying not to worry, trying to pray, and hoping that I would see my 65th birthday, my gaze landed on the wall calendar. It was Wednesday, July the 1st. My mother died on a Wednesday, July the 1st, 1992, at age 64. She, too, was hospitalized at the time. I didn't know it, but my daughter and two aunts were also watching their calendars and were as grateful and relieved as I when July the 2nd arrived. Irrational? Yes. I decided that Mom was watching over me. I was sure that God was.

On the 4th day, I was scheduled for an MRI of my brain. I had had MRI's before, and because of claustrophobia, I had required pre-medication. No one asked, and I was too ill to think of asking, so off I went to be encased in a tunnel. Since I was in a constant state of drowsiness if not fully asleep, I decided that keeping my eyes closed in the tunnel would be easy. All that I needed to complete my time in the MRI machine was a visualization to keep the panic at bay. A peaceful, comforting visualization. And someone to hold my hand. Jesus and I went into that tunnel together. His arms held me tightly, and we sang hymns: lovely, meditative Taize hymns, for the entire time. I was sad when that beautiful experience was over, and I believed that whatever the future held, I would be ok.

I was discharged home on July the 3rd in a wheelchair, with a walker for future use and with orders for in-home PT (physical therapy) and OT (occupational therapy). I was considered too weak to withstand inpatient rehabilitation due to the 3 hours of PT required daily and was also at risk for falls, so my family provided 24/7 monitoring for the first two weeks. I was discharged on full liquids with some pureed items due to the constant choking and the esophageal issues. By now, weight loss was another problem.

For the first time in my life, I experienced true vulnerability, and I didn't like it one bit. My physician was unable to give an estimated date of full recovery.

> *When we are no longer able to change a situation, we are challenged to change ourselves. Victor Frankl*

10

The First Year: July 2015-June 2016

Fall seven times, stand up eight. Japanese Proverb

Arriving home in a wheelchair was not only a humbling experience, but for someone who doesn't like to ask others for help, it was a prophecy of challenges to come. Fortunately, it was a small chair, because the main bathroom on the main floor is quite small. I became skilled at tiny 4-point turns, and the only damage to the house was some scuffing and loss of paint on the door and vanity.

The damage to the muscles of my upper body was another story. In straining and pushing my weakened, traumatized neuromuscular system in order to maneuver the wheelchair and transfer myself from the chair to the bed, the muscles spasms that began in the hospital soon increased to an excruciating level of pain. Heat, cold, medication — nothing brought relief. When trying to hold my head in an upright position, the pain was almost unbearable. In order to avoid triggering even more intense spasms, I literally rested my head on the bathroom countertop while sitting in the wheelchair as I brushed my teeth. When resting on the couch, my son would raise my head by lifting the pillow beneath me. I have never known such agony! In desperation one night, my daughter called my friend, a massage therapist, for advice and suggestions. After two home visits (yes, home visits!) and several sessions with a portable TENS unit, the pain finally began to subside and continued to improve over the next four weeks.

Sometime during these early days, my ability to hear would often disappear or be distorted. When my auditory nerve finally decided to settle down, I was left with a slight hearing impairment in my left ear and tinnitus in both ears. On good days, the tinnitus sounded like a soft symphony of crickets chirping, but on others, the sound could resemble the whine of a leaf blower or dentistry drill. Annoying, but it seemed minor in comparison to what had happened to the rest of my body.

The next month was an exhausting and often frustrating blur of trying to adjust to a different way of life. Even when my family was with me, I wore my cell phone like a heavy necklace in a camera case around my neck. I would not consider a lifeline. This was temporary!

My daughter brought me her stair step exercise equipment so that I could easily sit in the tub and use a hand-held shower. On days when I was too tired to shower, I discovered that disposable bath cloths were wonderful inventions! I would not consider a transfer tub chair. This was temporary!

The full liquid diet would continue until I had a normal swallow study, and liquid nutritional supplements were the brunt of my diet. I tried not to read the labels but couldn't help myself. Full of ingredients that I couldn't pronounce, they did have the calories and protein that my body needed to survive. I now weighed 93 pounds and needed energy to heal and to do my physical therapy.

Without my daughter, I am convinced that I would have starved! She must have made me gallons of her homemade mashed potatoes that were the consistency of thick, potato soup and "chicken shakes" that were a heavenly mix of stewed chicken, seasonings, and broth. This was blenderized so that I could drink it a through a straw.

Don't make a face until you try it, and until you've had nothing but sweet, liquid nutrition for weeks! Along with a small container of baby food fruit, this wonderful, satisfying meal was my supper for 6 weeks, and I never tired of it! My husband or son would heat and serve this flavorful combination each evening, and it felt like Thanksgiving! The liquid supplements were breakfast and lunch, and I discovered a new addiction: frozen yogurt—especially pistachio and, of course, cake batter! My anti-inflammatory diet was demolished, but I was grateful to be able to swallow and for a family that loved me.

I would tire very easily, and I would sleep after every effort. A shower, eating, taking a phone call, having a visitor, therapy—all were followed by a deep sleep. When the physical or occupational therapists would leave, I would be asleep before they got to their car.

I initially called the physical and occupational therapists the "parade of strangers." They seemed to wander daily in and out of my home with their resistance bands, waist belts, and ideas for awakening and strengthening my damaged nerves and muscles. They told me that had I not been in excellent physical condition and been on the healthy anti-inflammatory diet for the years preceding this event, I may not have walked again...or even lived.

As they encouraged and applauded every baby step that I made, I quickly came to call them my cheerleaders. I put beads on a string, took steps with a walker, and graduated to walking in the grass and doing one minute at a speed of one mile per hour on the treadmill with their support. In case of a fire, I learned how to get myself outside to safety. To their repetitions of "you are as tough as nails—you can do this," I must have done what felt like hundreds of modified squats from my couch. I used my piano to attempt to restore feeling and finger coordination in my hands. Most importantly, my therapists allowed me to use what was meaningful to me to develop my treatment plan.

One day in particular is embedded permanently in my memory. It was early in the rehabilitation process, and I had my ballet pictures scattered around the house to remind others — and myself — that this person in the wheelchair was not who I am.

My therapist asked me to tell her about ballet and the exercise class that I taught in my parish nurse ministry, so I told her about my years of dancing and the Mind, Body, & Spirit class. She then suggested that we try something different, something that I had developed muscle memory for, to stimulate the neuromuscular system.

My husband and I had previously turned an extra bedroom into a space where my piano, ballet barre, and my favorite books lived. My therapist rolled my wheelchair into this room and stopped several feet in front of the ballet barre and mirrored wall. She helped me stand and placed my hands on the barre. After selecting one of my favorite CD's, she started the music, and said, "Now, teach me your class. If you need it, the chair is right behind you."

My movements were not strong, fluid, or particularly graceful, but they were movements that my body knew, and they were correct. The tears were flowing down my face and hers as she said, "This is how you will get stronger, and we will build from here." And that day, I again prayed through plies.

> *...As decades of my muscle memory engage,*
> *Rhythmic ritual becomes a meditation,*

Focus sharpens to a stillpoint,
And I pray through pliés....

Get-well cards from family, friends, co-workers, and the congregations of both my home church and the church where I worked as a parish nurse filled my mailbox every day. Facebook messages and calls brightened my spirits.

In spite of the support and progress, I began to experience anxiety, especially about my future. A sense of depersonalization pervaded: it seemed as though the world outside of my home continued, but I was no longer a part of it. Although I have always loved being at home and having some time alone, this was too much. All was surreal, the walls were closing in on me, and I couldn't stop any of it. Some days were dark, and the feelings even darker. I tried to hide these feelings from my family. They had been so frightened when I was hospitalized and remained quite concerned. I didn't want to add additional worry, but I'm sure that they probably knew.

I tried to focus on gratitude, but the efforts felt false and superficial. I tried to find joy. My mother used to say, "Just go through the motions." So I went through the motions until I could hear the message.

Sometimes that message seemed to come from our cat, JB. JB had adopted us 14 years previously. We had just moved into a new home and saw what seemed to be some stray kittens in the woods nearby. Like apparitions of white and orange, they would appear briefly near the creek and then disappear for days.

A week passed. It was a hot day, and I decided to water the plants on the front porch. As I opened the front door, I glanced towards the porch swing. Curled into a ball on the swing cushion, a small white and orange cat was watching me. I expected her to leap down and run for the woods, but she didn't move. I sat on the porch floor and softly called to her. She did leap down, but much to my surprise, she ran towards me and landed in my lap! She was mostly white with large patches of orange scattered across her small frame. The second surprise was that she only had part of her tail! There was no sign of injury, and she appeared to have been born that way. As I talked to her, she began to "talk" back, and that's when I got the next surprise: this cat didn't meow, she quacked! Literally quacked—like a duck! Her beautiful green eyes looked at me with trust, and it was almost as if she knew me—that she recognized me. Maybe, she did.

Eight years before, I met another small, white and orange cat. She was dumped at a facility where I worked as a supervisor. She was sweet and gentle, and the entire staff loved her. And fed her, of course. One morning I arrived at work to find that she had been injured by a car. Her tail had been crushed. Wrapping her securely in a towel, I carried her to the veterinarian's office next door.

As I walked in, dogs of all sizes began to bark and howl in the waiting room. The cat managed to get one tiny paw free, and the disaster began! Terror turned this small, gentle creature into a wildcat fighting for her life. In trying to escape both the dogs and me, she clawed her way across my chest, neck, and face until she arrived at the top of my head. I managed to get my hands around her. Convinced that my plan was to toss her in the middle of the dogs, she dug her claws into my scalp and began to bite my fingers repeatedly. The veterinarian and his assistant were finally able to contain her. They called animal control and sent me to the emergency room. Someone called my husband to meet me there. When he saw me, he thought I had been in a car wreck. Blood was pouring across my face and down my chest. My hands were already swelling.

At home, I worried about this little cat. It wasn't her fault. She had been terrified. She was a sweet and gentle little soul who would probably be euthanized. After her quarantine time passed and there was no evidence of rabies, I drove to the pound. When I told them that I wanted to get her out of jail, they thought I was crazy. They knew the story. I filled out the forms, and they put her in my carrier. They then handed me a ticket for failing to have my cat vaccinated! "But she isn't my cat," I exclaimed. They replied "She is now. You have two days to get her vaccinated." With her purring her thanks from the back seat, I took her immediately to my vet. The office needed her name to register her. "Jail Bird. Just call her Jail Bird." Although the doctor said that her tail was seriously injured and may need to be amputated at some point, we were still able to find Jail Bird a loving home.

This new, little cat curled contentedly in my lap, and looking at me like a long-lost friend, she bore a startling resemblance to Jail Bird. They were almost identical. The only difference was the tail. A perfect, healthy little half-tail. Is this possible? Could she possibly be…? Mysterious and puzzling phenomena do occur, so who am I to say what is possible or not? All I know is that she seemed to know me, and, and looking back, I believe she did recognize me. We named her JB — short for Jail Bird, of course. And she moved into our home and hearts.

JB was unique. Remember, she had been abandoned and, like the ugly duckling, was born with only half of a tail and a quack instead of a meow. She understood the dark days. An adorable, sweet, and sometimes annoyingly needy cat, she was my husband's almost from the beginning. She liked me, but she adored him! When my world changed, so did our relationship. When I was alone, with only my thoughts to keep me company, she was there. She began to spend her days curled on the couch with me, and we became the best of friends. JB, Jail Bird, whoever this little being was, became my therapy cat. Her presence, her purring, and even her bizarre quacking seemed to quieten the constant ringing in my ears and relieve the anxiety and darkness in my soul. She took good care of me, and I grew to love her dearly.

I was approved for my short-term disability benefits from my employer and read for the first time the words "disabled-you are unable to perform your current job at this time." This benefit was provided for up to six months at which time I would need to apply for long-term disability benefits. Six months? Surely, I would be back at work long before six months!

As the days and weeks passed, my instinct told me that, as much as possible, I needed to return to my healthy diet. Could nutrition work its miracle a third time? I would keep my tasty chicken and beef shakes, my creamed white potatoes, and the delicious frozen yogurt that brought me joy and smiles, but how could I ingest my healthy vegetables and fruits in a raw or frozen state without additives or sugar with this full-liquid diet? The answer came to me immediately: smoothies! As soon as I was strong enough to use my walker to stand alone and take a few steps, I began to experiment with the blender and combinations of real food: real food that met my criteria! Remember these three?

- Is this good fuel?

- Does it have good nutritional value?
- Is it healing?

Some of my smoothies had odd combinations of ingredients. My family would make awful faces when they heard what was in my glass but usually liked these special smoothies after trying a few sips. After the motor died from overwork in my old blender, I researched how to layer the ingredients and how much liquid should be added. Most of my smoothies had either frozen or ripe bananas for a creamy texture and natural sweetening. One smoothie consisted of canned pumpkin, ginger, cinnamon, honey, and soymilk. Another had peanut or almond butter, soymilk, and frozen banana slices. Two of the smoothies quickly became my favorites, and several family members even requested them! My "blue ribbon winner" was my breakfast smoothie that had vegetables, fruit, protein powder, and, sometimes plain Greek yogurt.

This was my "eat the rainbow" meal for the day! For the vegetables, I would use kale, spinach, carrots, broccoli, cucumber, or frozen beets. Along with the banana, the fruits used were usually strawberries, blueberries, peaches, raspberries, or dark cherries. I could almost hear my body say, "thank you!" when I drank one! In second place was my favorite "dessert" smoothie: a delicious concoction of cocoa powder, nut milk, banana, and frozen blueberries. I also experimented with making batches of the smoothies and freezing each serving in a mason jar. This worked beautifully! My nutrition was finally back on track!

Six weeks passed. After developing a comprehensive plan for self-directed therapy and exercise which involved 10-20 minutes of work done twice daily, I graduated from in-home physical therapy. With the encouragement of my physical therapists and home health nurse, I made a formal complaint with the FDA about my experience with Levaquin.

The sensation of touch and the reflexes in my legs and arms were diminished, so my driving was restricted. When someone was with me, I could now drive short distances in low traffic and at low speeds. During my first attempt, my husband drove us to an empty church parking lot. Then it was time for me to practice. Having 48 years of driving experience offered no reassurance as I painstakingly adjusted to how the steering wheel, brake and gas pedals felt to my tingling hands and feet. After 5 minutes, my legs and brain were tired, but I finally managed one smooth lap around the parking lot.

I had a repeat swallow study done, and although there was still some weakness present, I could return gradually to a normal diet. While this was exciting, some foods were still difficult to swallow. I continued to have my smoothies at least once daily. They had become my food of choice! At this point in my recovery, I also added CoQ10 and a quality probiotic supplement to the B vitamins and magnesium that I had taken from the beginning. The medical equipment company came to collect the wheelchair. My sense of vulnerability rose for a moment, but then I happily waved good-bye!

The months passed. The card ministry continued in earnest. Hundreds of cards and messages later, I am convinced that these messages of love and healing "prayed me well."

I gradually began to tolerate more solid foods and, for the most part, followed my anti-inflammatory diet. But I remembered my earlier insight: life is short. Some foods are simply good for the soul, and I enjoyed those foods several times a week and on any special occasion!

My hands and feet no longer hurt, but felt numb, like I had gloves and socks on them. Each morning when I awakened, I would gingerly move my fingers and then my toes. Were the gloves and socks gone? Did they feel normal? Could I even remember what normal felt like?

I continued my twice daily exercise regime of light weight work, balance work, gentle ballet barre, core strengthening, and the treadmill. I also included Mind, Body, & Spirit routine on days when I was able. Since pliés are scattered throughout, I found that the gratitude flowed in a continuous stream as this joyful movement sent a loving and healing message to my body and soul. I added repetitions, time, and distance on the treadmill. I had difficulty with uneven surfaces or inclines, so walking outside was difficult. I still slept frequently during the day and always had to rest after the exercise sessions. I could drive alone but still with restrictions, so I added 30 minutes of water yoga weekly and swimming 6 laps on a separate day to my therapy plan.

Having made a small amount of progress, I felt it was time to venture out of the house. Dea took me to Target to shop, and my legs lasted about 20 minutes. That included the walk to and from the car! Other friends would take me along with them to the library or the grocery store. Again, I was good for about 20 minutes. I never knew how wonderful grocery carts were for support, and I wished that I could have squeezed into the child seat! The next "field trip" was to a shopping center 60 miles from home. My daughter drove me, and we had such a good time talking that I was already tired by the time we arrived. We shopped in several stores and, after several minutes in the last one, I couldn't remember where we were. It was time to go home!

For my next advancement up the ladder of normalcy, my daughter excitedly invited one of my friends from another state to visit with me for the weekend. She thought it would bring needed joy and life into my four walls and, in normal circumstances, I would have been thrilled! Panic and dread consumed me as the thought of having to stay awake, alert, and follow a thread of conversation for longer than a few minutes almost suffocated me. I know that I disappointed them, but I was practically incoherent by the time I was able to help them understand.

What I now recognize as depression occurred several months later. I had continued to have some dark times, but November 2015 was like an explosion of loss and overwhelming grief. I had a follow-up visit with my doctor. My reflexes were no longer diminished. They were absent. I had none. When I asked when I could expect to recover, he told me that I would probably know what damage was permanent in several years. January 2017 was the date he gave.

Two more years. Was my recovery sliding backwards? My defenses started to crumble.

When I got home, I did what had always worked when life knocked me down. I went to my ballet barre. I prayed through plies. The tears flowed. I called Rev. Michael Bailey, the pastor of First Presbyterian Church where I was still listed as their parish nurse and tried to tell him that I didn't know when or if I could return to work. He and I had worked closely together for almost 10 years, and he knew me well. Concerned, he drove 30 miles to deliver a "lucky" bamboo plant, a message of hope, and most importantly, his ministry of presence to comfort me. His message for me was to embrace the lessons the darkness will teach, and that God would be with me in those moments in ways not possible in the sunny times!

Several days later, I learned from my husband that my cousin's breast cancer had metastasized to her bones and lungs. She asked him to tell me because she just couldn't bear to give me that message. She had Stage IV metastatic cancer.

Dea was more than just my cousin. Along with our grandmother, our mothers, aunts, uncles, and my dad, we grew up in the same home. Older than I by 10 years, Dea helped my mother care for me when I was born, and she never quit caring for me. As adults, we became the best of friends, and we shared life's joys and sorrows, our losses, and our laughter. Both of us nurses, we were each other's first call when life or health crises happened. When I had been hospitalized, she had visited each day and informed me that I was not going first, not leaving her here alone. Pointing out the wheelchair by my bed, I told her that she was already the last one standing. She did not find that funny, but my laughter was contagious, and we laughed together as we thought we would for many years to come.

Metastasis. What an ugly, prophetic word. I went to her home immediately. So much love. So many tears. She said that I was her rock, but I knew that she was mine. I didn't know what I would do without her. We both had reminded each other hundreds of times over the years to "Rejoice Always!", but words now failed us. Darkness settled in my heart.

In late December, my short-term disability benefit ended, and the long-term disability was approved. Because my employment status ended when the long-term disability was approved, the healthcare organization that covered my benefits while employed at First Presbyterian terminated my position. Once again, the staff and congregation supported me and decided to retain me as their parish nurse, and once again, Michael brought words of comfort. "Regardless of your 'status,' you are a beloved child of God. Nothing can change that—bask in that truth today and every day." Cards, calls, and visits continued, but thoughts of gratitude and spirituality were suffering.

Rev. Karla Woggan, the priest at the Episcopal Church of the Ascension, my home church, visited me regularly. I shared with her that my relationship with God and my gratitude practice were struggling. I was trying to hear what God was saying to me—trying to discern what He wanted me to do with this grief and with my life. She said something quite simple, yet profound, that washed like a river of peace over me. She said that when you feel you can't hear God's voice, listen for Him in the voices, in the words, of those who love you. I listened, and the voices were unfailingly filled with hope and love.

Those voices eventually became God's, and as I listened, I discovered something about my relationship with the Holy Trinity. I dutifully recited "in the name of the Father, the Son, and the Holy Spirit" as part of the liturgy as I had been taught, but my perception and understanding of the Trinity was vague to say the least. I realized with surprise that it was God to whom I had prayed and called upon for my entire life, and I had no idea why. It became very important—an obsession, actually—for me to fully grasp this concept in a way that made sense to me. For the Trinity to mean more than words I regularly chanted. I was in a spiritual crisis, and somehow this seemed to be the key that would unlock my confusion. I needed my relationship with God to be whole. I needed consecration.

Immersed in the sacred mysteries and riddles of the unknown, I found myself returning again and again to my concept of wholeness, transformation, and my early mantra of praying through pliés. I thought of darkness and of light. An idea began to form, but it was only when I remembered the MRI—that frightening tunnel with Jesus as my companion— that the key began to turn. By opening the rusted areas of my mind that had been unused and neglected, I was able to let go of concepts and theology that simply did not resonate with my vision or experience. A revelation was released, and I finally knew what the Holy Trinity meant to me:

Thank you, God, for creating me, and loving me completely.
Thank you, God, for the Father, who blesses me,
 For the Holy Spirit who guides me and lights the fire within,
And for Jesus, who holds my hand.

Early in 2017, I attended my first ballet class since Levaquin. My ballet home welcomed me with the love and the encouragement found in decades of friendship. My confidence and my steps were hesitant, but with hand on the barre, my muscle memory responded. When the barre work was complete, we moved to the middle of the floor for center work. There was no barre or support here. It seemed as if the floor began rapidly expanding in all directions, flowing outward until I felt like I was standing alone in a space at least the size of football field! Alone, with nothing and no one to support me.

With my pulse racing, I inched carefully back toward the barre and continued the center choreography knowing that I could reach the barre if needed. Because balance was an issue—I often tilted towards the left without realizing it—I learned to use the mirror to tell me where I was and in what position.

In February, we learned that JB was dying. For one month, I became my little therapy cat's hospice nurse. I rubbed comfort medications on her ears and tried without success to find soft food that she could eat. She hardly "quacked" anymore and seemed to find comfort only when we were holding her. In March, her vet made a special trip to our home, and I held JB as I kissed her goodbye. Rejoicing…always.

By the end of March, my condition had not improved, and I felt that I was keeping the church in limbo. A decision needed to be made. My last official day as a parish nurse was April 24, 2016. A reception and celebration of my ministry there was held in my honor, and I have never felt as surrounded by love as I did that day. It was a day of great joy, gratitude, and loss, and as my husband and I drove away with the contents of my office surrounded by baskets of flowers, I knew that God had blessed me when he led me to that sacred place. God loved me and would continue to do so. His light would pierce the darkness.

As I had for most of my life, I continued to find joy in ballet. I attended class when I was able, and my confidence slowly grew. In May of 2016, I was able to do a very simple waltz in the ballet, The Wizard of Oz, because my sweet grandson agreed to be my partner! Years before, and at his request, we had waltzed before. I knew my partner! Six feet tall and quite strong, he held my arm and waist and gently guided me through our choreography. There was no chance he would let me fall!

May today there be peace within. May you trust God that you are exactly where you are meant to be. May you not forget the infinite possibilities that are born of faith. May you use those gifts that you have received, and pass on the love that has been given to you. May you be content knowing you are a child of God. Let this presence settle into your bones, and allow your soul the freedom to sing, dance, praise and love. It is there for each and every one of us.   St. Theresa of Avila

11

The Second Year: June 2016-June 2017

What would it be like if you lived each day, each breath, as a work of art in progress? Imagine that you are a Masterpiece unfolding every second of every day, a work of art taking form with every breath. Thomas Crum

One year has passed, and it was a long and challenging year. It was a year of losses as well as blessings. While I made progress, it had been slow, and I was told that it could be years — or never — before full recovery occurred. I still dealt with peripheral neuropathy that affected sensory, motor, and autonomic nerves. My hands still felt as if I were wearing gloves; my feet, socks. While I regained a good deal of muscular strength, my stamina was still poor, and when I was tired, neither my legs, my balance, nor my brain seemed to work very well. My legs often felt very heavy and wobbly, like jello, and I still had difficulty walking on uneven surfaces. Poor stamina and fatigue were major issues and, when fatigued, my concentration was impaired. There were brief episodes of unusual visual problems: it would suddenly seem as if I were looking through red, green, or blue colored lenses. Disconcerting, but fortunately, these only continued for a period of several weeks before disappearing! I still had no reflexes in my legs, feet, and arms, so I walked a little differently and continued to have driving restrictions: 5 miles, low traffic, and low speed.

My doctor was concerned that the neuropathy might be progressive. The autonomic nervous system appeared to be damaged. My blood pressure and heart rate were erratic: orthostatic hypotension, a condition where one's blood pressure would drop drastically upon standing, became quite concerning. For example, it might drop to 68/40 or 74/51. I learned to sit or lie down quickly to avoid fainting. I also learned that there is risk for the development of neurodegenerative disorders such as Parkinson's, Multiple Sclerosis, or ALS after having a severe neurotoxic reaction.

I continued with a variety of exercises and physical therapy regimes that PT designed for and with me. I exercised every morning and evening for approximately 20-30 minutes each, and I still rested afterwards.

I progressed to where I only rested three or four times during the day instead of actually sleeping for hours every afternoon! I tried to do a variety of things that stimulated nerves, muscles, fine motor skills, and neuron regeneration including water yoga, lap swimming, walking on uneven surfaces, piano exercises, brain games, strength training with weights and resistance bands and, of course, my ballet barre.

During this year, I volunteered from home with an organization called the Quinolone Vigilance Foundation, an organization that seeks to educate healthcare providers and the public about fluoroquinolone antibiotics while advocating for victims, supporting research efforts, and presenting to the FDA, to representatives in Washington, and the Centers for Disease Control.

Dea and I talked daily and visited whenever we were able. We treasured our time together and were grateful that

God's hand had pushed us to make even more time for each other.

In January of 2015, six months before Levaquin and metastasis entered our worlds, Dea had called me after filling in her calendar for the upcoming year. Although we had always gotten together for special occasions and called each other regularly, we both had very active lives. She said that as she looked at her filled day planner, she saw bridge clubs, circle meetings, and lunch dates. She then said that she realized she had scheduled time for everything and everyone except for someone who meant the world to her — me. We decided to make time for us, and that included frequent lunches and visits. I worked 25 miles away then as a parish nurse, but she would drive there to have lunch several times a month. We would get together locally for lunch or a visit on days that I didn't work. These days of early 2015 were special days that gave us the gift of time and memories...memories that would keep us warm during the winters of our lives that were just beyond the horizon.

As this one-year anniversary passed, my husband and I bravely decided to take a risk. It was a huge leap of faith! We decided to take our trip to Yellowstone and the Tetons. We also decided to add four other National Parks: Bryce Canyon; Arches; Canyonland; and Zion. In mid-August, fortified with boxes of food, water, seasonal clothing, bear spray, and my trekking poles, we began our adventure, and my husband drove the entire round-trip, over 7800 miles, while I either slept or gazed out of the window. As we visited the parks, I would sometimes wait in the car while he captured thousands of digital memories.

Several times, I stayed in our motel room and slept during the afternoons. We made sure that I rested, because I was a long way from home. Fortunately, many incredible sights were visible from our car or within short walks! Bryce Canyon's mysterious and magical columns called hoodoos, the magnificent, yet delicate-appearing arches of Arches National Park, Zion's soaring massive sandstone cliffs of pink and red that soar into the sky as they narrow into slot canyons, and Canyonland's barren moonscape were all easily seen. The Tetons were as breathtaking as I remembered, and we remained in the shelter of their towering peaks for 4 days.

Yellowstone, however, will always hold a special place in my heart and deserved more than a phrase or a sentence. Its siren call also demanded that I do more than watch from the window or take a short walk. Lower Falls is a waterfall, a 300-foot-high torrent of water that has carved the Grand Canyon of Yellowstone. Rainbows arch across the mist that rises beneath it. Lower Falls was the reason we had wanted to return to Yellowstone. This trip, we saw Lower Falls from all viewpoints, including one that required walking down, and then back up, a curving metal stairway of 328 steps. My trekking poles gave me the equivalent of 2 good legs! Resting along the way, it took hours to accomplish, but I did it! I could not, would not, waste this opportunity!

The topography and landscape change around every turn of Yellowstone, a geological wonder of over 2 million acres that has been evolving for millions of years. Above the Yellowstone River and the icy Yellowstone Lake, waterfalls roar, and thermal mouths belch steam that fill the air with odor of sulphur. Massive boulders deposited during an ice age, the turquoise abyss of boiling prismatic pools, geysers exploding toward the sky, bubbling mud pots, and the peaceful quiet of the Lamar Valley are all mere pieces of the whole that is Yellowstone. When traveling through this strange and mesmerizing world, with its chaos and its beauty, it is as if you are traveling and experiencing the timeline of God's creation!

We returned home in mid-September, and a new cat, Boo, joined our family. Boo, a beautiful, long-haired muted calico, was a stray who had appeared at my daughter's home years before. She had spent most of her time outdoors until one of the family's dogs decided to terrorize her. Traumatized, she then began hiding in the basement. After moving in with us, she seemed to quickly leave the scary memories behind. Bringing light and laughter to each day, she morphed into a funny, affectionate little clown. She began greeting me early each morning. As soon as she heard my morning music, she would bound into my ballet room and watch as I began my Easy 8's. When I moved on to my floor stretches, she would either lie beside me or hop onto my stomach to help me! During my prayers, she would rest quietly, and after we ate breakfast, she would sleep for the rest of the morning. She had as many routines as her human mom!

Like the previous November, November of 2016 brought darkness and grief. On November the 26th, Dea died. Over the years, we had found ourselves at the bedsides of our loved ones, holding their hands and each other's during their final moments as we prayed our grandmother, my mother, her mother, and my dad to heaven. While my physical and emotional health were still fragile, I was where I wanted to be, where I must be — at her bedside, holding her hand, praying her to heaven. The last one standing. Rejoicing…always.

On December the 8th, my birthday, the snow began falling. Huge, lovely flakes fell from early afternoon until late that night. The world became a white canvas, and where Christmas lights adorned the trees and shrubbery, multi-colored lights glowing through the blanket of snow created prisms of color. It had never snowed on my birthday before, and I was enthralled! Dea had loved snow, and I found myself waiting for her excited voice, calling to tell me to look outside! Instead, it was her daughter-in-law who called. Her sweet and thoughtful words made this rare and breathtaking beauty complete: "Look outside! Dea never missed your birthday, and this must be her present to you!"

January 2017 arrived: two years since my doctor said that it would be two years before I knew the severity of the neurological damage and what it meant for my long-term prognosis. Since very little had changed since the beginning of my second year, I tried to keep my focus on what I had accomplished and on what I intended to accomplish.

As part of my New Year's resolutions during this milestone month, I decided on a plan to stimulate and strengthen my brain connections. In Chapter 6 on Stress and Relaxation, I described my decades-old morning routine. This included starting my day by reading something beautiful or inspirational. My 2017 resolution was to deepen and expand these morning readings. I added educational books to my variety of reading materials, and I made an intentional effort to learn and memorize something new each morning. Since my goal was to actually study the material, I could only read several pages daily without losing my focus. My capacity to learn grew, and the desire to learn more about some of the ideas and content found me frequently "googling" in order to learn even more! An avid reader since childhood, fiction works had been my preferred genre until this new yearning for knowledge became a morning addiction. Not only did it help my brain, I enjoyed it so much that I have read several of the books 2 or 3 times!

As the brain connections became stronger, I began to think seriously about writing my book. Through the late winter and spring, I would jot down ideas as they occurred, but it was much more difficult than memorizing words that someone else had written!

A close friend, Betty, who suffered from a serious, chronic disease called granulomatosis with polyangiitis,L visited throughout this year. We had lovely, healing times together. Betty and I spread our yoga mats in my ballet room, turned on some beautiful music, and did some simple ballet steps followed by floor stretches. I then led us through healing visualizations, and we prayed. Both of us discovered that on those days, we could remember the joy of dancing! We could remember what normal was — even if it was only for one hour. After the first time together, I texted Rev. Bailey at First Presbyterian. "I have been a parish nurse again! It was only one hour, but I was a parish nurse today!"

In February, I was able to return to First Presbyterian to lead my Mind, Body, & Spirit class. As I got stronger, this group of women had even offered to come to my home or to drive me from my town to theirs so that our class could continue. Their confidence in me and my love for them inspired me to take a chance! The first class was so obviously exhausting that one dear friend invited me to her home for lunch and a nap before attempting the drive home. I waited until I got home for both, and I was determined to continue my class.

There were still dark days, even dark months, when I felt depersonalized, living in a twilight zone where I didn't really exist, where my mind felt as numb as my legs. Days that the world kept turning, but I was not moving with it. Days that the walls closed in. Days of sadness, of grief when losses seemed to outnumber the blessings. And days of anger, when I imagined the FDA imploding and sharp, lethal shards piercing the armor of pharmaceutical negligence and greed.

Lupus is a gentle companion in comparison. Almost as if it knew my body could handle no more, lupus has been quiet since Levaquin entered the picture. I can embrace lupus. I can shower it with love and gratitude. Because it is part of me, my immune system, my own cells. Levaquin was different. This was an alien entity that poisoned my neuromuscular system, leaving some pathways feeling like ground zero. While I was grateful for the progress made and the blessings I had received, there was no gratitude toward this enemy. This was war. I didn't want this to define me, to color how I saw the world, but it was not easy. It literally cloaked me like Peter Pan's wayward shadow. I felt its presence with every step, with the electrical currents that stabbed occasionally through my feet, with ripping-like pain in my tendons, with every glass that I dropped, with every quiet moment that now rang in my ears. On days when the walls closed in, I was aware. Even in sleep, it frequently tormented me. My dreams were filled with situations in which I couldn't walk, I couldn't function. Unconscious reminders that reinforced loss and an unknown future thereby undoing the day's progress and gratitude work. I was different. And so was my world.

Walk on, through the wind
Walk on, through the rain
Though your dreams be tossed and blown.

Walk on, walk on, with hope in your heart
And you'll never walk alone!
lyrics from "Carousel" by Rodgers & Hammerstein

12

The Third Year: June 2017-June 2018

My barn having burned down, I can now see the moon.
Mizuta Masahide (17th century Japanese poet and samurai)

Two years have now passed. I may be different, but this would not be my story. Frequently, I heard my mother saying, "do not give in, you have my strength, it has always been in you." I worked hard to "reinvent" myself. Along with my exercise/therapy regimen, I wrote several hours each day during this year, and I finished my book! On June the 13th, I received notice that my book was approved for publication. I was elated! It was the first time I felt that I had accomplished something meaningful since Levaquin, and I wanted to celebrate this date.

My eyes landed on a devotional book that I hadn't read in many years titled <u>Jesus Calling</u>, by Sarah Young. <u>Jesus Calling</u> is a devotional that does not give a year, only the month and day so that it can be used over the years. The devotions are written as if Jesus is speaking personally to you. I read the devotion for June the 13th.

"I am creating something new in you: a bubbling spring of joy that spills over into others' lives. Do not mistake this Joy for your own or try to take credit for it in any way. Instead, watch in delight as My Spirit flows through you to bless others. Let yourself become a reservoir of the Spirit's fruit.

> *Your part is to live close to Me open to all that I am doing in you. Don't try to control the streaming of My Spirit through you. Just keep focusing on Me as we walk through this day together. Enjoy My Presence, which permeates you with Love, Joy and Peace."*

As I finished those words, I realized that exactly 2 years earlier, on June 13, 2015, I took the first dose of Levaquin. Goosebumps covered my arms. With the realization that this message applied to that day in 2015 with just as much significance as they did on this day in 2017, I read them again.

> *"I am creating something new in you…Your part is to live close to Me, open to all that I am doing in you… Just keep focusing on Me as we walk through this day together."*

And I rejoiced, as peace and closure began to settle in my soul.

I began to give copies of my book to a few friends, and I was anxious to hear their opinions. Betty, my companion in healing, excitedly took her copy. Several days later, we met for lunch. We talked about having healing groups and the Mind, Body, & Spirit class at her new studio. It was a beautiful space, and we made delightful plans!

On July 18, 2017 Betty died after a sudden flare of her illness. She had such a beautiful spirit and was a blessing to her family and many friends. There are still times, when Mind, Body, & Spirit and I practice alone in my ballet room, that I hear her laughter in the music. And see her smiles as she moves with me. Rejoicing…always.

Although I had written <u>Praying Through Pliés</u> as therapy for myself and for my family and close friends, my book began to find an audience. People bought extra copies to give as gifts, and strangers would contact me asking me about my experience and how it related to theirs. No one was more surprised than I was!

I was asked to do my first presentation. Public speaking had always terrified me, and one of my first thoughts when I had to leave my career was that at least I never had to speak in public again. God had other plans!

Perhaps I still had a purpose, and perhaps that is why He helped me write this book. If He has given my book wings and opened a door for me, how could I say no? I agreed to do the presentation, and more importantly, I decided that when doors opened, I would walk through them!

My physical symptoms and condition reached a plateau during this third year—I had seen no progress in the last 6 months of this year. Although I could drive more than 5 miles now, my reflexes, initially "diminished" have been " totally unresponsive for almost 3 years, so I still drove at low speeds and in light traffic. Most likely due to autonomic nervous system damage, my blood pressure and heart rate remained erratic at times. The crickets chirped loudly in my ears. The peripheral neuropathy in my hands, feet, and legs is unchanged. Balance remained a challenge. While my muscles were stronger, stamina remained poor. My body was like a faulty alternator or a battery that simply wouldn't hold its charge. Because my legs and my brain still did not function very well when I was tired or stressed, I still required frequent rest periods throughout the day. While my brain exercises have helped, my ability to multi-task, problem solve, and focus remained challenged. Adding studying and memorizing new material daily was an important addition to my daily exercise and writing commitment. Sometimes, I would still try to remember what "normal" felt like, and I realized that this was my new "normal." I turned 67 during this year, so I supposed that I must be retired.

As this year came to a close, gratitude remained the foundation of my health practices and my life. Joy and beauty unfailingly lifted my heart, and I searched for them daily. Some lovely music, my morning readings, a few minutes of stretching, and meditative breathing while listening for God's daily whisper began my days. Whatever the days held, they ended with "Rejoice Always, in everything give thanks!"

I tried to practice gratitude and to remember my many blessings in every moment of every day: I can walk without assistance — I can even do a little ballet! After all, I danced with my oldest grandson! I was able to be there to see him graduate with honors and see two beautiful ballerina granddaughters perform! In May, I had the privilege of being in the ballet, Sleeping Beauty, alongside my granddaughters! Being the queen, I was basically a stage prop, but I felt a part of every step of the ballet. I have seen my other two grandchildren excel in basketball, baseball, and their schoolwork. The bunny pajama pants from my oldest granddaughter, a little stuffed, red fox from my childhood that was brought out of hiding by my youngest granddaughter, and the hand-made cards from my other granddaughter and grandson all brought love and comfort while I was hospitalized, and they continue to do so. My daughter has continued to nurture and applaud every step of progress, and my son has called every day. He would search the news for funny animal stories for me to enjoy. I have had a brilliant and caring physician who not only recognized what had happened to me and took immediate steps to support my nervous system but who continues to support and believe in me! I continue to lead my Mind, Body, & Spirit class one hour each week at First Presbyterian Church. Wonderful friends have been there for me. My incredible husband has been not only a constant pillar of love and strength, but a pillow where I rested both my head and my heart. He and my entire family have been steadfast in their support, have tolerated my "down" days, and have never given up hope for a full recovery. Many have held me in their prayers. I am blessed.

At the end of year 3, I returned to the barre, that place where pliés transition dance — and my life — from one step to the next. The music and the dance called my name, and my mother's strength lifted my eyes heavenward. And I prayed through pliés.

...Prayers filled with gratitude
To all who have made this moment possible,
Thanking God and my body
For one more time at the barre...

"I believe deeply that God does his best work in our lives during times of great heartbreak and loss, and I believe that much of that rich work is done by the hands of people who love us, who dive into the wreckage with us and show us who God is, over and over and over. Let yourself fall open... to anticipation, to the belief that what is empty will be filled, what is broken will be repaired, and what is lost can always be found, no matter how many times it's been lost." — Shauna Niequist, Bittersweet: Thoughts on Change, Grace, and Learning the Hard Way

13

The Fourth Year: June 2018-June 2019

Tell me, what is it you plan to do
with your one wild and precious life?
Mary Oliver

It has been 4 years since Levaquin, and time is now measured as pre-Levaquin and post-Levaquin. During the past four years, there have been times when there were more steps backward than forward, when loss, sadness, anger, depersonalization, and yes, depression tried to beat me. I won't deny that the dark days continue. Days when my toolbox of choosing my thoughts and perceptions and positively reframing the negative thoughts are challenged to the point where I am exhausted. And I fail. I fail because I am human, and I am reminded to be gentle with myself. I do believe, however, that I have become an expert at hiding these days from those that I love. On the days that my false smile is successful, an interesting paradox occurs: In hiding my brokenness from others, I have fooled myself as well, and I am whole once again!

Four years, and many questions remain. Is "my new normal" permanent? Will damaged nerves continue to regenerate? Can I hope for further improvement? Will the nerve cells deteriorate from the trauma? Will the disabling effects worsen?

In September of 2018, my high school class held its 50th

reunion. We celebrated the Hickory High School Class of '68 with style! It was a memorable weekend that was filled with the richness of renewing friendships. We played, we laughed, and we celebrated the importance of relationship. I had known most of my classmates for over 45 years, and some of my closest friends today were present! We celebrated how this group of children who became teens were a vital and significant part of the adults that we had become and how they also affected the paths that we chose to travel. I believe that every person we meet along the way changes us. I know that this special class had a huge impact on me. I also know that I treasured every moment, every hug, and every smile at this reunion, and I was grateful that I was able to attend.

On the good days, I had been attending an adult beginning ballet class since the early fall. It was often a struggle, and my steps would falter quickly as my effort increased. My technique was poor at best. In February of 2019, I began class as usual, but I became aware within minutes that something had shifted. My technique was sound, and my stamina, although still poor, did let me move normally for several minutes! My teacher, who had been a close friend for almost 20 years, noticed and immediately asked if I wanted to be in the ballet in June. Her confidence and enthusiasm were contagious. I was terrified, but a door had opened, and I would walk through it. I knew what it would take to make the choreography part of my muscle memory — part of my brain connections. I made a personal promise to myself to practice the steps daily. In the privacy of my ballet room, over and over again, I coaxed damaged neurons as I prayed through pliés.

My primary care doctor, who had provided such excellent and compassionate care, left his practice in May 2019, to become a full-time hospitalist. During this year and shortly before he left, my Social Security Disability application was finally approved. After 3 years of multiple denials and appeals, and numerous forms and letters that my doctor completed, it was finally over. After a judicial hearing that was distasteful, confrontational, and even degrading, it was approved. Without the incredible support I received from this doctor, it would not have happened.

At our last appointment, I was feeling vulnerable and anxious. How can I continue to beat the odds? I asked him what I could do to lessen my chances of developing a neurodegenerative disorder. Always guiding and encouraging me on this journey, he offered parting advice.

> *"Keep doing what you're doing. Continue your healthy lifestyle.*
> *Research everything that you encounter, including medications, foods, insecticides, herbicides, and cleansers, and avoid it if it has the potential for adverse effects on the nervous system.*
> *If you need surgery, be careful with anesthesia. Your diaphragm was damaged along with your autonomic nervous system. The surgeon and anesthesiologist need to know this.*
> *Avoid getting sick. Your antibiotics are limited. After a severe neurotoxic reaction to an antibiotic, you may have a similar reaction to others.*
> *Avoid getting cancer. Chemotherapy drugs often cause neuropathy and neurological side effects."*

Avoid getting sick? Avoid cancer? I'll do my best! Although we laughed, I knew he was serious. He also told me he would not forget me and would think of me often. While reminding colleagues that didn't take the fluoroquinolone warnings seriously, he would think of me. And do his best to educate both them and his patients. Do I miss him? Yes! He was an integral part of my battle armor! Am I grateful that he was there when I needed him the most? Yes! Every day. Beyond grateful. Rejoicing…always.

I have worked hard physically, mentally, emotionally, and spiritually. I continue to work on personal reinvention. I now lead my Mind, Body, & Spirit class several times weekly. Requests for presentations, or inspirational speaking engagements, are becoming more frequent, and I completed a certification course in Etherapy to expand my counseling licensure. The ability to counsel online and from home is an exciting concept and possibility for my future!

My neurologist calls me a walking miracle, and most days, at least on the days that I rest frequently, I would agree. The peripheral neuropathy remains. I no longer wiggle my toes and fingers to check for socks and gloves, because like the ear crickets, or tinnitus, they apparently are permanent residents. While my muscle strength continues to improve, stamina has not. Reflexes are still nonexistent.

My brain can still embarrass and frustrate me as I search for words or put words together that make no sense. During this year, as I have tried to stimulate and push my brain's ability to think, focus, and learn, I have also experienced something I have heard referred to as brain fatigue. It is difficult to explain, but my brain gets tired! Like a computer when it freezes from having too many windows or programs open, my brain simply shuts down. For me, this is different from the word searching or confusion mentioned earlier. I appear to be awake, but my eyes aren't really seeing, and my brain quits processing information. I haven't rested enough and, at this point, nothing restores my mental functioning except sleep.

The autonomic neuropathy is not only limiting and frustrating, it can be downright dangerous with its plummeting blood pressure drops. It's not always convenient to stand slowly and stay near something that I can grab as I sink to the floor! Also, part of the autonomic system misbehaving is another disturbing phenomenon. Experiencing a common emotion such as anxiety, anger, or joy very intensely can occasionally trigger a spike in blood pressure accompanied by a pounding heartbeat, facial flushing, and a horrific, sudden head pain that feels as if my head will literally explode. Fortunately, this doesn't happen often, and except for several days of scalp soreness, the symptoms usually disappear within 30 minutes.

Yoga, an important part of my early rehabilitation, has become an important part of maintaining the health of my mind, body, and spirit. Research confirms that yoga is beneficial for stress, depression, balance issues, anxiety, the joints, bones, muscles, heart, and brain. After learning that it is also healing for the nervous system, especially the autonomic nervous system, I began to practice yoga regularly.

Each day, I have fought for health, and in looking back, it seems that I have for most of my adult life. I have learned, however, along with the benefits of positive thinking, gratitude, exercise, nutrition, rest, and the managing of stress, that love is the greatest healer. Both love received and love given. I have also learned that perhaps fighting for health is too aggressive of a stance to take. I no longer fight or do battle with this body that I have been given to care for, this body that has allowed me to live, to love, to work, and to dance. Instead, I now treat my body tenderly and with no small amount of respect. I try to give it what it needs to stay healthy, but I also remember my earlier epiphany that life is short, and tomorrow is not guaranteed. So, I enjoy that piece of cake. And lick the bowl that held the batter. It feeds my soul.

Thinking about gratitude and blessings reminds me of something important — the message from Chapter 2 about being grateful to lupus and all it had to teach me. I am reminded, as I write about Levaquin, that if I had not practiced the healthy lifestyle that I learned from living with lupus, that I might not be here today to tell this story. The disciplines of exercise, diet, rest, and faith not only kept lupus from destroying me, they truly enriched my life and strengthened my mind, body, and spirit. They enabled me to survive the war that Levaquin declared on my body, and when the initial battle was over, their practice provided the framework and the motivation for recovery and rehabilitation.

Living with a chronic disease can be challenging and overwhelming, but the practice of gratitude can be transforming. I can truly say that I am grateful to a disease called lupus. I could even say that it may have saved my life!

But Levaquin? Let's just say that rejoicing has not come easily or quickly. Following the initial anger and rage, came the stage I choose to call "because of Levaquin."

Because of Levaquin, I've had time to write, and while I have always appreciated my husband, my appreciation has grown into a firm belief that my husband is the greatest man on this earth!

The evolution of my perception of Levaquin has taken years, and it remains a work in progress. Choosing to permanently reframe my experience with Levaquin into something positive may take a lifetime. We may even send a colony to Mars before it is completed.

I do know that 4 years post-Levaquin, on unexpected and unremarkable days, I can whisper "I am grateful to Levaquin." I choose to be grateful to Levaquin during those moments, not for what it has cost me, but because of what it has given me. Levaquin rocketed into my life and when I was ready, slowly revealed its gift. It unwrapped before me the gift of time, reinforcing that I must make every moment count, and the gift of making both my days and my relationships richer than I could ever imagine.

I am grateful for so many blessings found in every moment and every year. My husband, family, and friends have walked this road with me without hesitation and continue to cheer me on my journey. My heart is full of their love for me—and mine for them. I can walk and dance! I can eat—and eat with joy! I saw Yellowstone again and the Tetons breathtaking majesty at sunrise!

My morning routines continue to begin my days—and Boo's—with grace. Those readings have provided continuing improvement in both my memory and my mental focus, and I believe that they helped me write a book! And that little book has opened unexpected doors and given me the courage to walk through them! My book brought some extraordinary and delightful people into my life while also giving me the opportunity to renew old friendships!

I wrote a book that grew wings—wings that carry its message of healing, gratitude, and faith. A book whose message has allowed me to still be a parish nurse. A book that can share with others the power of praying through pliés.

———

In June of 2019, I danced again! Really danced. In a ballet. On a stage. With no one physically supporting me. Without a mirror to tell me whether I was upright—or beginning to fall. Sharing a stage again with granddaughters whose smiles were louder than any applause! Sharing a stage with granddaughters whose pink tulle swirled across my arms and face as they floated gracefully by me. Around me. Before me. Their hands gently grazing mine in an elegant, lovely, and surreal world of Tchaikovsky and shimmering tulle. These were the enchanting, magical moments of Act I, and as I watched regally from my chair as a member of the royal court, I breathed it all into the fabric of my heart, mind, and soul. Into a special place where treasured memories shine brightly. Like shimmering tulle. Forever.

Then the curtains closed, and the lights went down. It was time for Act II. It was time for my dance, a four-minute dance with friends who had supported and encouraged me. A dance in honor of my husband, my family, and my friends, some of whom were in the audience. A dance in memory of those who were not.

In that dark space and with heart pounding, my old performance anxiety tried to surface, but I took a deep breath and remembered how I had gotten there. I smiled. My whole being smiled! And when the curtain opened and the lights illuminated the darkness, I stepped out on to that stage, and I danced. Rejoicing always…praying through a thousand pliés!

Darkness deserves gratitude. It is the alleluia point at which we learn to understand that all growth does not take place in the sunlight! Joan D. Chittister

Epilogue

There are two ways to live your life. One is as though nothing is a miracle. The other is as though everything is a miracle. Albert Einstein

Writing the 1st edition of this book did not come easily; in fact, it was quite difficult. As I previously mentioned, the outline, poem, and early pages of the first half of this book that described my journey with lupus had been completed for some time. I was busy with family, working, and dancing and had little time to write. After Levaquin's devastation, the urge to return to writing as part of reinventing myself became even stronger. I felt that I needed to combine these two parts of my journey, but the ideas just wouldn't come together. I had kept a diary of sorts and did Facebook updates for my friends, so I had the facts. I just couldn't seem to connect my notes into an organized flow describing what had happened to me. Even more challenging was how to bring the two parts together in a way that would be understandable and meaningful. I continue to deal with a variety of neurological issues, and my brain no longer worked as well as it did prior to June of 2015. Once an efficient multi-tasker, I now had problems with focus, concentration, and organization of information. I simply could not connect the ideas that formed the foundation of my journey. Frustrated, I was ready to abandon the whole idea, but then something miraculous happened. My mother helped me finish my book.

I have always experienced vivid dreams, but these dreams were like no others. My mother was standing in front of me, smiling and welcoming me with open arms.

"You can always come bunk with me. I have missed you so much and would love for you to be with me, but you have something that you need to do."

I awakened thinking, "bunk with me?" I knew what it meant but had never used this term or even heard it in years. What did she mean? The next night, she returned.

"Finish your book. Your story should be told. Our story should be told. I will help you."

She visited my dreams for four nights. She spoke no more but smiled and nodded her encouragement. Her love enveloped my sleep and spilled into my days.

The words began to fill me, and I began to write. I would write until I was exhausted each day. I didn't want to stop for fear that the words would stop flowing, or that I could no longer put them together. But the words continued to come, and in three weeks, this book, our story, was finished.

This is how the 1st edition, called Praying Through Pliés, was completed, and it was published in June of 2015. Two years have passed since that publication—four years since Levaquin.

As I began to write my 2nd edition, I re-read <u>Praying Through Pliés</u>. Errors seemed to jump from the page that I had not noticed before. Misspellings, long, confusing sentences, chronological mistakes, and more were stunning reminders of the trauma my brain had suffered and of how I had struggled to write my book. I sent my brain a hug and a "thank you," and told myself that it was ok. Those errors were only confirmation of my message, a message that was heartfelt, true, and exactly what I had meant to say.

Physically and mentally, I am stronger. Stronger, but still lacking in stamina. Without resting throughout the day, the endurance needed to function normally and productively is absent. Damaged neurons falter. I stumble, and my thoughts become disorganized.

Writing this 2nd edition has been equally difficult. Why equally difficult, since my thought processes have improved markedly? The answer is twofold. I have learned that exercising my brain by writing or by concentrating causes my brain to feel as tired as my legs feel after attempting a one-hour ballet class. The thoughts begin to disconnect, and some disappear altogether. The errors make their way onto the pages. I then know it's time to rest again.

Also, without rest, it is more difficult to hear my other muse — my mother's voice from that still-vivid dream. If I rest as I should, my thoughts begin to flow, and her message still resonates in my mind, and I hear her words again:

"Finish your book...I will help you."

The memory of her love and her strength continues to be my inspiration; her nightly visits and her words, the fuel for my words. Although this 2nd edition is finished, my journey, and therefore hers, will continue. I may never know if God spoke through my mother, or my mother, through God, but I do know that they were both with me as I wrote. And both God and my mother will remain beside me, just as they have always been, and will continue to be.

...Slow, lovely notes flow.
My eyes glance heavenward,
I am mindful only of this moment,
And I pray through pliés.

Fluoroquinolone Antibiotics:The Facts

Fluoroquinolone antibiotics such as Levaquin, Cipro, and Avelox, have been in the news with increasing frequency in recent years. While awareness is growing about adverse reactions to this class of drugs, there remain doubt and lack of knowledge among healthcare providers and the general public. Fluoroquinolone antibiotics are approved to treat certain bacterial infections and have been used for more than 30 years. They work by killing or stopping the growth of bacteria that can cause illness. Without treatment, some infections can spread and lead to serious health problems.

Fluoroquinolones were designed to treat anthrax, plague, and severe life-threatening infections—not urinary tract infections, sinusitis, and bronchitis. These drugs are neurotoxic and may cause widespread, permanent damage to the nervous system. They can affect the central nervous system, the brain, and peripheral nerves. They also have the potential to damage and destroy connective tissue such as the tissue found in muscles and tendons. They can attach to DNA, cause hearing loss, and disrupt the mitochondria, which are the power houses of cells. Memory and concentration issues, psychiatric problems such as depression, severe anxiety, hallucinations, and even suicides are linked to these antibiotics. There are reported deaths and permanent disabilities. These reactions can begin after one dose or many, and may be apparent immediately or days, weeks, months, or in some cases, years later.

The FDA reports 3,000 deaths and over 200,000 complaints from fluoroquinolone antibiotics. Dr. Charles Bennett, a hematologist and researcher at the Medical University of South Carolina, says that because only 1% of victims ever file a complaint with the FDA, the number of deaths is probably closer to 300,000. Also a researcher with SONAR, The Southern Network on Adverse Reactions, Dr. Bennett references an increased rate of the later development of neurodegenerative diseases such as ALS, MS, and Parkinson's in patients who have suffered a neurotoxic reaction to fluoroquinolones. On September 11, 2014, Bennett filed a petition with the FDA calling on the federal agency to change the drug labels to better warn patients of the risks.

- The FDA issued its first black box warning in **2008** regarding the possibility of tendon injury or rupture.
- In **2013**, another black box warning was issued stating that permanent nerve damage such as peripheral neuropathy could occur.
- A warning in **May of 2016** sent to internal medicine practices, family practices, and pharmacists advised that serious side effects associated with fluoroquinolone antibiotics generally outweigh the benefits for patients with sinusitis, bronchitis, and uncomplicated urinary tract infections who have other treatment options. The warning continued by stating that these antibiotics are associated with disabling and potentially permanent serious side effects that can occur together and can involve the

tendons, muscles, joints, nerves, and central nervous system.

- A new warning from **May of 2017** expands on these symptoms and states that side effects have been documented for up to 9 years after the initial reaction.

- July 10, 2018: The U.S. Food and Drug Administration began requiring safety labeling changes for a class of antibiotics called fluoroquinolones to strengthen the warnings about the risks of mental health side effects and serious blood sugar disturbances and make these warnings more consistent across the labeling for all fluoroquinolones taken by mouth or given by injection. "The use of fluoroquinolones has a place in the treatment of serious bacterial infections—such as certain types of bacterial pneumonia — where the benefits of these drugs outweigh the risks, and they should remain available as a therapeutic option. The FDA remains committed to keeping the risk information about these products current and comprehensive to ensure that health care providers and patients consider the risks and benefits of fluoroquinolones and make an informed decision about their use," said Edward Cox, M.D., director of the Office of Antimicrobial Products in the FDA's Center for Drug Evaluation and Research. There are more than 60 generic versions. The safety labeling changes the FDA is requiring today were based on a comprehensive review of the FDA's adverse event reports and case reports published in medical literature. The new class-wide labeling changes will require that the mental health side effects be listed separately from other central nervous system side effects and be consistent across the labeling of the fluoroquinolone class. The mental health side effects to be included in the labeling across all the fluoroquinolones are disturbances in attention, disorientation, agitation, nervousness, memory impairment and delirium. Additionally, the recent FDA review found instances of hypoglycemic coma where users of fluoroquinolones experienced hypoglycemia.

- **July 17, 2018**: Amid safety concerns, the makers of a popular antibiotic have halted production on the drug. Janssen pharmaceutical companies of Johnson & Johnson discontinued production of the oral and IV versions of Levaquin in December 2017. However, Levaquin may still be available in pharmacies until 2020. Also discontinued was the production of Floxin Otic ear drops, another fluoroquinolone. Dr. Charles Bennett, with the Southern Network on Adverse Reactions (SONAR), and who is referenced earlier in this article, said that Janssen's decision will have little impact on public safety because other drug makers are still making the generic form, known as levofloxacin.

- Dec 20, 2018: A U.S. Food and Drug Administration (FDA) review found that fluoroquinolone antibiotics can increase the occurrence of rare but serious events of ruptures or tears in the main artery of the body, called the aorta. These tears, called aortic dissections, are ruptures of an aortic aneurysm that can lead to dangerous bleeding or even death. They can occur with fluoroquinolones for systemic use given by mouth or through an injection. Fluoroquinolones should not be used in patients at increased risk unless there are no other treatment options available. People at increased risk include those with a history of blockages or aneurysms (abnormal bulges) of the aorta or other blood vessels, high blood pressure, certain genetic disorders that involve blood vessel changes, and the elderly.

- **September 2019:** Dr. Bennett has filed a petition with the FDA, asking that doctors who prescribe fluoroquinolones require patients to sign a release that they understand the risks before taking the drugs. Despite the FDA black box warnings, detailed warnings are buried deeply within a 35-page drug information insert. He gave suicides as an example. The FDA reported that 174 suicides have been tied to this medication in the past 20 years and made the following statement to a news agency: "The FDA is reviewing the petition and will respond directly to the petitioner. It is important that health care providers and patients are aware of both the risks and benefits of fluoroquinolones and make an informed decision about their use. For some serious bacterial infections, including bacterial pneumonia among others, the benefits of fluoroquinolones outweigh the risks and it is appropriate for these antibacterial drugs to remain available as a therapeutic option. More information about fluoroquinolones can be found on FDA's web site." The FDA could take more than a year to decide on Dr. Bennett's request.

If you have an adverse reaction to any medication, please report it to the FDA through their MedWatch online link!

Living a Healthy Lifestyle

[9] Do you not know that your bodies are temples of the Holy Spirit, who is in you, whom you have received from God? You are not your own; [20] you were bought at a price. Therefore honor God with your bodies. 1 Corinthians 6:19-20 (NIV)

Do you honor God with your body and treat it as a temple? If not, why? There are many excuses and sometimes legitimate reasons why living a healthy lifestyle is difficult! Life itself can be reason enough sometimes! Even making small changes can be beneficial. As you look at the following areas, read and re-read the quotes, and then take an honest assessment of your life. Each category has its own chapter in this book. Review the simple suggestions. Try to list two changes in each area that will make a positive impact on your health and commit to trying them for two weeks. You may find yourself wanting to add more!

Exercise

If exercise could be packed into a pill, it would be the single most widely prescribed and beneficial medicine in the nation.
Dr. Robert Butler, founder of the National Institute on Aging

1.
2.

<u>Sleep</u>

And if tonight my soul may find her peace in sleep, and sink in good oblivion, and in the morning wake like a new opened flower then I have been dipped again in God, and new created.

D.H. Lawrence

1.
2.

<u>Stress and Relaxation</u>

"It's not stress that kills us, it is our reaction to it." Hans Selye

1.
2.

<u>Nutrition</u>

The doctor of the future will no longer treat the human frame with drugs, but rather will cure and prevent disease with nutrition."
Thomas Edison

1.
2.

Choices and Gratitude

Everything can be taken from a man but one thing: the last of the human freedoms – to choose one's attitude in any given set of circumstances, to choose one's own way.   Victor Frankl

Are your thoughts healthy or destructive? How do you normally face illness, challenges, or loss? Will you <u>choose</u> helplessness, anger, embracing the struggle, or gratitude?

The following shows examples from the book on reframing negative thoughts to positive ones. Try to remember negative thoughts you have had in the past week, month, or year. How did they affect your mood or behavior? How could you have re-framed them into a positive thought?

Negative Thought	Positive Thought
I can no longer hike in the mountains.	I can walk.
I miss my once active social life.	I am grateful that my best friend called today.

Gratitude Journaling

If the only prayer you ever say in your entire life is thank you, it will be enough. Meister Eckhart

If you haven't already begun a daily gratitude practice, promise yourself that you will begin now! Your gratitude journal is ready for you to start! Simply list 5 things for which you are grateful. Tomorrow, list 5 things as you begin your day and 5 things before you go to bed. Repeat daily and be prepared for your life to change!

1.
2.
3.
4.
5.

"Can you see the holiness in those things you take for granted–a paved road or a washing machine? If you concentrate on finding what is good in every situation, you will discover that your life will suddenly be filled with gratitude, a feeling that nurtures the soul." Rabbi Harold Kushner

Rejoice

Rejoice always, in everything, give thanks!
1 Thessalonians 5:16,18

What does this scripture mean to you?

Have there been circumstances where you found it difficult to "Rejoice Always?"

Have there been circumstances where you found it impossible to "Rejoice Always?"

Are there circumstances that could possibly occur in your own or other's lives where you can't imagine being able to "Rejoice Always?"

What has helped you to "Rejoice always", **and in everything**, give thanks?

Miracles

"There are two ways to live your life. One is as though nothing is a miracle. The other is as though everything is a miracle." Albert Einstein

What does this quote say to you, and how do you live your life?

How do you define a miracle? Must it be an extraordinary, unexplainable event or simply an important and perhaps life-changing occurrence?

Have you experienced a miracle or seen one occur in someone else's life?

If so, how has your life and perspective changed as a result?

Finding Your Pliés

You have read what pliés mean in my life. What are your pliés, and how can you discover that special state of being where your wholeness lives? Begin by asking yourself the following questions, and put down everything that comes to mind:

As a child, what places did you love, and what did you enjoy doing?

What places or activities now bring you joy and peace?

What calls you and where do you return, even if it's only in your mind, when you are stressed, anxious, or need comforting?

From these answers, notice if anything resonates with you. Are there any themes that re-occur?

Why is the answer even important for you? Why is finding your special state of being, your pliés, so vital to your well-being?

Praying through pliés is where transformation begins for me. This foundational, flexible step in ballet makes it possible to transition from one step to the next, both in dance and in my life. In order to reinvent and transform ourselves during times of illness, loss, difficulty, or simply because you want to improve your life, you must transition — you must find your own pliés.

This is your challenge, to find your pliés, that place where you can remember what normal is. That place where your own reinvention and transformation can happen. That place where you will recognize with peace, joy, and gratitude that health and healing don't always mean that there is absence of disease. Be it in prayer or meditation, yoga, running, listening to music, or hiking to the brink of a waterfall, search within yourself and find your answer.

May your journey towards transformation and wholeness
be blessed,
and
May you rejoice, always!

The Morning Readings

As requested by readers, I have provided a simple, chronological listing of the books and readings that have expanded my mind and my world since January 2017 — over a thousand mornings! There are thousands of pages represented here and note that an asterisk indicates the books that have been read more than once.

The Natural Parks: America's Best Idea by Dayton Duncan & Ken Burns *

Mindfulness: The New Science of Health & Happiness published by Time Magazine as a special edition

Principles of Meditation: Eastern Wisdom for the Western Mind by Simpkins & Simpkins

Sabbath: Finding Rest, Renewal, and Delight in our Busy Lives by Wayne Muller*

The Atlas of Mysterious Places: The World's Unexplained Sacred Sites, Symbolic Landscapes, Ancient Cities

An Illustrated World History: Prehistory and The Ancient World — a series by McRae Publishing for Sandy Creek and Barnes & Noble *

Into The Blue by Virginia McKenna of the Born Free Foundation

The Soul of an Indian and Other Writings from Ohiyesa (Charles Alexander Eastman) edited by Kent Nerburn

<u>Great Smoky Mountains National Park</u> by Ken Jenkins and Carson Brewer

<u>The Blue Zones: Lessons for Living Longer</u> by Dan Buettner with National Geographic

<u>The Blue Zones Solution: Eating & Living Like the World's Healthiest People</u> by Dan Buettner with National Geographic

<u>The Blue Zones of Happiness</u> by Dan Buettner with National Geographic

<u>Wild Planet</u> published by the Natural History Museum

<u>Meditations of John Muir: Nature's Temple</u> by Chris Highland

<u>A Journey with Luke: The 50 Day Bible Challenge</u> edited by Marek Zabriskie

<u>The Complete Idiot's Guide to Music History</u> by Michael Miller *

<u>A Journey with Acts: The 50 Day Bible Challenge</u> edited by Marek Zabriskie

<u>Aging as a Spiritual Practice</u> by Lewis Richmond *

<u>The Gift of Years</u> by Joan Chittister *

<u>History Year by Year</u> published by the Smithsonian *

<u>Living Buddha, Living Christ</u> by Thich Nhat Hanh

<u>A Thousand Mornings</u> — the poetry of Mary Oliver

<u>Stardust: The Cosmic Recycling of Stars, Planets, and People</u> by John and Mary Gribbin *

<u>The Gnostic Gospels</u> by Elaine Pagels

<u>How, Then, Shall We Live: Four Simple Questions That Reveal the Beauty and Meaning of Our Lives</u> by Wayne Muller *

<u>Atlas of the Civil War: A Comprehensive Guide to the Tactics and Terrain of Battle</u> by Neil Kagan and Stephen Hyslop for National Geographic

About the Author

The author is a Registered Nurse with over 35 years of experience. She has also held certification in psychiatric and mental health nursing and has been a Licensed Professional Counselor (LPC) in the state of North Carolina for over 20 years. She and her husband share 3 children, 5 grandchildren, and a cat, Boo. She has studied ballet since the age of 5, was a competitive swimmer and swim team coach, and enjoys playing the piano and traveling.

Surviving Lupus, Levaquin, and Life, the 2nd and expanded edition of Praying Through Pliés, is the author's true and inspiring journey of living for decades with a chronic, autoimmune disease and then surviving a devastating and disabling neurotoxic reaction to the fluoroquinolone antibiotic, Levaquin, in 2015.

Visit her website at www.rhondajeanbolton.com to leave comments on her blog, to send an email, and to learn about her books, her programs, and her services. Available for inspirational speaking and Etherapy, an online counseling service, she may be contacted for scheduling through her website. Updates on videos of the Easy 8's and the Mind, Body, & Spirit class will also be posted!

<u>Reviews for Praying Through Pliés</u>

the 1st edition and prequel to <u>Surviving Lupus, Levaquin, and Life!</u> received unanimous 5-Star ratings on Amazon! Readers are saying:

…a beautiful book about surviving and thriving despite challenges. While it is about lupus and an "ordinary" antibiotic that caused life-changing---and life-threatening--side effects, I recommend Praying Through Plies to anyone dealing with a chronic illness…with practical tips for healthy eating, sleeping, and managing life's complexities and maintaining a positive mindset, no matter what. It's short, simple and a pleasure to read so it makes a wonderful, caring gift for just about anybody facing illness or physical limitations…

…this book has made me want to change my life…Her spirit and determination are beyond words. I was jolted by the information about antibiotics and how some of these can destroy your body and maybe even your life. This book lifted my spirits and I am determined to follow her suggestions… This is going to be my new go to give away book for my friends and family...

…beautiful…heartfelt…warms your soul…I can't imagine how difficult it was to relive in order to bring hope to others…an inspiration for how to live one's life… Sandy Barton, BS, PTA

…a book that anyone and everyone in the medical community especially should read… Thank you for writing this very important book…

…It is a testament to the author's courage, tenacity and indomitable spirit. Read it in an hour and come away with a lifetime of insights on how nutrition, exercise and faith can help one cope with some of life's most formidable challenges…

…a blessing to read this book and begin applying within my life…

...this book will bring hope and peace and a will to fight through whatever comes one's way...

...a masterpiece of transformation...

...A wonderful true story of courage and strength! It has something for everyone wanting to improve their health and lives as well as important information about how antibiotics can adversely affect your body. Encouraging and informative...

...Beautifully written and accurately written about the class of antibiotics called fluoroquinolones. I highly recommend anyone who wants to save themselves and their health to read this true account of what happened to this author. I know you will love it as much as I do...

...This book describes, not only living through Lupus, but dealing with the horrid effects of this drug and the courage it took to survive it all...a remarkable book that I recommend to everyone...it teaches us so much we need to know and to spread the word about this dangerous type of drug and the courage to overcome it — with God's help, many, many prayers, the love of her family and friends, and the fortitude it took on her part to overcome...

A wonderful true story of courage and strength! It has something for everyone wanting to improve their health and lives as well as important information about how antibiotics can adversely affect your body. Encouraging and informative.

...Eloquent realism...Resonated with me. A joyous look at chronic illness and how to return to living. A life full of gratitude and hope.

Writer's Digest Awards 2018
Judge's Commentary on <u>Praying Through Pliés</u>

...a unique, amazing book about the author's unique, amazing journey. I appreciate this author...her spirit...her attitude... it's clear that the author cares very much about her readers... a lovely, inspiring book filled with faith, hope, and love. I hope it is read by millions...

131

www.ingramcontent.com/pod-product-compliance
Lightning Source LLC
Chambersburg PA
CBHW061812250726

48657CB00001B/398